Values-Based Leadership in Healthcare

Sara Miller McCune founded SAGE Publishing in 1965 to support the dissemination of usable knowledge and educate a global community. SAGE publishes more than 1000 journals and over 800 new books each year, spanning a wide range of subject areas. Our growing selection of library products includes archives, data, case studies and video. SAGE remains majority owned by our founder and after her lifetime will become owned by a charitable trust that secures the company's continued independence.

Los Angeles | London | New Delhi | Singapore | Washington DC | Melbourne

Values-Based Leadership in Healthcare

Congruent Leadership Explored

David Stanley

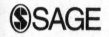

Los Angeles | London | New Delhi
Singapore | Washington DC | Melbourne

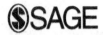

Los Angeles | London | New Delhi
Singapore | Washington DC | Melbourne

SAGE Publications Ltd
1 Oliver's Yard
55 City Road
London EC1Y 1SP

SAGE Publications Inc.
2455 Teller Road
Thousand Oaks, California 91320

SAGE Publications India Pvt Ltd
B 1/I 1 Mohan Cooperative Industrial Area
Mathura Road
New Delhi 110 044

SAGE Publications Asia-Pacific Pte Ltd
3 Church Street
#10-04 Samsung Hub
Singapore 049483

Editor: Donna Goddard
Assistant Editor: Jade Grogan
Production editor: Tanya Szwarnowska
Copyeditor: Peter Williams
Proofreader: Rosie McDonald
Indexer: Cathy Heath
Marketing manager: George Kimble
Cover design: Wendy Scott
Typeset by: C&M Digitals (P) Ltd, Chennai, India
Printed and bound in Great Britain by Ashford
Colour Press Ltd

© David Stanley 2019

First published 2019

Apart from any fair dealing for the purposes of research or
private study, or criticism or review, as permitted under the
Copyright, Designs and Patents Act, 1988, this publication
may be reproduced, stored or transmitted in any form, or
by any means, only with the prior permission in writing of
the publishers, or in the case of reprographic reproduction,
in accordance with the terms of licences issued by
the Copyright Licensing Agency. Enquiries concerning
reproduction outside those terms should be sent to the
publishers.

Library of Congress Control Number: 2018963082

British Library Cataloguing in Publication data

A catalogue record for this book is available from
the British Library

ISBN 978-1-5264-8764-3
ISBN 978-1-5264-8763-6 (pbk)

CONTENTS

ABOUT THE AUTHOR

David was born in Liverpool, England, and grew up in Whyalla, South Australia. He trained as a nurse at the Whyalla and District Hospital. His career has been eclectic and diverse and after becoming a midwife he taught midwifery as a volunteer in Zimbabwe, later moving to the UK where he coordinated Children's Services in York. He also became a Nurse Practitioner in Worcestershire before undertaking a nursing doctorate at Nottingham University. David's doctoral research was in the area of clinical leadership, and he has continued to investigate how clinical leadership and nursing leadership are perceived and practised. On completion of his doctorate, David returned to Australia to continue his academic career. He has supported a number of nursing students on international practice trips to Thailand, Tanzania and The Philippines. David continues to work in academia, researching and writing about nursing and clinical leadership, teaching nursing and leadership principles and supporting and educating the future nursing workforce.

FOREWORD

One of the wonderful aspects of a career in healthcare is the chance to be exposed to leaders across a range of disciplines and contexts. David Stanley and I have been colleagues in clinical and management roles over many years, working to support the growth of education and training opportunities in developing countries. David has been a leader in nursing and academia, challenging historical concepts of leadership and exploring how other models, such as Congruent Leadership, may be used in the future to ensure leaders can drive improvements in the healthcare system, benefitting patients and the community.

Values-Based Leadership in Healthcare: Congruent Leadership Explored provides wonderful examples across many sectors, from leaders and scenarios that are immediately transferable to healthcare. Interesting and diverse role models guide students' understanding of how leadership styles can be translated at a personal and professional level. The breadth of different types of leadership theories covered provide a foundation for exploring the suite of traits and styles that contribute to the establishment of values-based leadership. From this the reader can consider and explore the concept of Congruent Leadership, an emerging model of leadership in healthcare.

Dr Stanley provides an opportunity to challenge prior leadership constructs, allowing us to reassess the best theoretical frameworks and models applicable to healthcare. It is an approach which promises to serve how healthcare leaders support and lead colleagues, in the hope that they in turn can shape and improve healthcare delivery.

Catherine Stoddart

PREFACE

Your beliefs become your thoughts

Your thoughts become your words

Your words become your actions

Your actions become your habits

Your habits become your values

Your values become your identity

Mahatma Gandhi, Indian politician and father of modern India

'LET'S START AT THE VERY BEGINNING'

Oscar Hammerstein II, the lyricist in the team of Richard Rogers and Oscar Hammerstein II who developed the musical *The Sound of Music* (and other musicals), had the character of Maria sing:

Let's start at the very beginning

A very good place to start

When you read you begin with ABC

When you sing you begin with Do, Re, Me.

Great advice, but when you picked up this book about values-based leadership you might be wondering if there are three easy steps to follow to help develop a leadership approach that is based on values. There are three, but there are also more than three. Nothing as complex as learning to read or sing or develop an insight into leadership is really as simple as three easy steps. The fantasy world of musical theatre is delightful but seldom realistic.

The topic of Congruent Leadership, a values-based approach to leadership at the heart of this book, is, however, relatively simple and, some might conclude, as simple as ABC or Do, Re, Me. However, there is a story that goes with it and it would make sense to start at the very beginning. Therefore, in this short prelude to this book, I aim to offer an outline of how the theory of Congruent Leadership was developed and how it may be used to help you become a successful or effective leader in your area of practice, your workplace, your organisation or your professional discipline, or indeed in any area of your life where you wish to develop a more values-centric style of leadership.

THE STORY

In the beginning: Indeed, throughout my professional career I have been a nurse. I started my nurse training (for training it was) at the Whyalla and District Hospital in 1980.

I was not encouraged to think too much beyond an acceptance of the established rules, along with not being encouraged to think for myself. I was not even allowed or encouraged to talk with doctors (who were portrayed as 'God-like' and remote from lowly nurses). Any new ideas, thoughts for change or even aspirations to leadership positions were positively discouraged. We were taught to be concrete thinkers and, as such, we were to be seen to do and not be heard. But things rapidly changed. At the start of my training all senior registered nurses (we called them 'Sisters' then) were addressed by their surname, but at the end of it we could call them by their first name. Also, caps, which were a common piece of attire linked to status and identity at the start of my training, had been abolished by the end of it. Radical stuff at the time and a sure sign that the health and nursing world was turning on its head.

When I completed my three years as a student nurse at Whyalla and District Hospital, I applied for and was lucky enough to secure a place on the Flinders Medical Centre Graduate Nurse programme. In 1984, this was a relatively new opportunity generally reserved for the new Diploma of Nursing students just emerging from college or university.

At Flinders Medical Centre I found myself part of a group of 18 university educated nurses (there was one other hospital-trained nurse in the intake of 20 'new grads'). I was placed on the orthopaedic ward for the first rotation of three months. I found myself well prepared for the hospital environment in comparison to the university-trained nurses. They seemed to lack both confidence and competence, they came late, missed handover, didn't know how to talk to patients, couldn't find their way around a medication trolley or the hospital, didn't know how a hospital worked, did not know anything about being a new 'Sister'. In short, I felt very disappointed with the direction nurse education was taking. These university-trained nurses were (I thought) 'poor' and compared to them I looked like a gift to the hospital workforce. I was slick, efficient and organised and felt very competent. In my three years at Whyalla and District Hospital I had been socialised into the nursing profession. I was the proud product of a structured, foundational concrete learning system and even though they didn't do things the Whyalla Hospital way, I soon learnt to adjust to the Flinders Medical Centre way.

However, by the time I had reached my final placement in Accident and Emergency something had changed. The 'university-educated' nurses, who just nine months earlier had their heads all over the place, were starting to 'run rings' around me. They would gather blood results and engage doctors in conversations about the results and even boldly make treatment suggestions that I wouldn't have dreamed of doing at this stage of my career. They were ahead of many of the junior doctors when it came to gathering observations and setting up for treatments and they were at home in the tearoom talking to any level of nurse and even other health professionals.

What had gone wrong? How had these graduate nurses become socialised so quickly? Was I simply not engaged in life-long learning? Had I even been learning or was I simply acting out the role I was taught at Whyalla Hospital?

It may have been some of these things, but after a long period of reflection (a very un-concrete learner thing to do), I realised that the university-trained nurses had learnt or been taught differently. They had been taught to think critically (not concretely), to approach clinical situations as problems to be solved. By their fourth ward rotation they had developed the registered nurse's role socialisation skills and skilfully employed their problem-solving, critical thinking skills, skills I was to learn were clearly vital to modern healthcare professionals. Like the lady sitting near Meg Ryan's character in the film *When Harry Met Sally*, I wanted what they had.

I soon saw that if I was to make nursing my career and if I was to progress as a professional nurse, I needed to re-learn how to learn and how to think like they did. I needed to become a critical thinker. I had other plans in the next few years and followed these up by doing my Midwifery training (again at Whyalla and District Hospital). Once this was complete I enrolled in a Diploma of Nursing and then a Bachelor of Nursing at Flinders University. I soaked up the education (for education it was). I was driven to learn and then practise critical thinking. It was very much up to me as a self-directed adult learner to map out my own learning journey and to navigate my way through the degree. It took some time to crack through my old concrete thinking ways, but by the time I had completed the Bachelor's degree, I had (I think) fathomed it out. I must have done something right, because I was awarded the Flinders University Medal for Health Science that year.

OK, I have gone a little off track here. However, my point is that I had finally realised that as a student nurse I had been trained not to think about things beyond what was expected and not to act beyond the role I was required to fill. The university-educated nurses I had met in 1984 and the education I had had while undertaking my diploma and degree had allowed me to recognise that only by thinking critically can we act differently, think differently and become leaders that can make change happen.

However, my journey with critical thinking was only just starting. It was not enough to know how to think differently. I also needed to shed some of the preconceived patterns and ways of behaving, or roles I had learnt as I was socialised into nursing. I also needed to learn something about confidence and the various ways of being a professional in the world of healthcare.

The next lessons came when I worked as a volunteer Midwifery Educator in Zimbabwe between 1994 and 1996. In Zimbabwe I worked with doctors in a completely different way. I was seen as an equal partner in the healthcare provision of the hospital, I was highly regarded for my midwifery knowledge, I taught myself how to do ultrasound scans and became an on-call nurse-anaesthetist, working with a primitive anaesthetic machine and with minimal medication. Mainly I supported the provision of caesarean sections and other surgery. I also assisted with minor surgery when the hospital was overflowing, drove the ambulance when the driver was not available and undertook midwifery practice that would be reserved for obstetricians in Australia such as delivering breech presentations and twins when no medical help could be secured, and having to deal with numerous complicated maternal and neonatal issues that in Australia were seen only very rarely. I left Africa both more confident and more practised in critical thinking.

From Africa, I travelled on to the UK and secured a number of senior positions including one as a nurse practitioner in a community hospital. This role was specifically focused on changing practice and building staff capacity for doing things differently. Having learnt to think critically and build my clinical confidence it was in the UK that I realised there was a third issue I needed to address in order to lead more effectively and support change. I needed to understand the process of change and how leaders could support or promote innovation and change. Without a clear plan or understanding of change, the likelihood of successfully implementing change was low.

I looked about for literature related to clinical leadership and found a plethora of information about leadership from a management perspective, but little about leadership for bedside, shopfloor, coalface leaders. So, I went back to study and completed a Master's of Health Science degree and then undertook and completed a Nursing Doctorate with my research focus on leadership. This provided hints towards the final keys to understand how values-based leadership can be used to become a more effective leader and support change and impact positively on quality and safe clinical practice.

Therefore, my three steps for developing an understanding of Congruent Leadership or a values-based leadership approach are:

1. Learn to learn effectively and develop critical thinking skills.
2. Become practised in applying values with confidence. And finally
3. Learn how to manage change and understand leadership and the process of supporting change.

What I learnt was that I did not need a big office, lofty title or leather chair to be a leader. I did not need to be a manager or get the biggest salary or have the most senior position. Leadership is so much more than managing or holding power. I learnt that leaders can make a difference simply by knowing what their values are and acting on them consistently. In this way, leaders can be anyone, at any level and in any position, simply by matching their values to the things they do, or having their values guide their actions so that others recognise them. The most fundamental type of grassroots and values-based leadership will result. Values-based leadership is different from other types or styles of leadership and it needs to be understood in a way that is different from other leadership approaches.

It has taken almost my whole career to work this out and it has involved years of research, reflection and reasoning. Of course, there are more than three steps for understanding values-based leadership or Congruent Leadership and this is where the rest of this book will help. Therefore read on and explore the full scope of these realisations in the remainder of this book. The content of each chapter is outlined below.

LEADERSHIP BACKGROUND:

CHAPTER 1: LEADERSHIP: WHAT WE KNOW NOW

This chapter outlines a number of theories that help explain what leadership is and how it can be understood. A range of leadership theories are described and used to precede a platform for understanding where Congruent Leadership theory fits with what is already known about leadership.

CONGRUENT LEADERSHIP OUTLINED

CHAPTER 2: CONGRUENT LEADERSHIP THEORY

This chapter elaborates upon the theory of Congruent Leadership. It describes what it means, how it is defined and what it constitutes. The chapter also highlights how Congruent Leadership is related to power, quality processes, innovation and change, why it offers a solid foundation for leaders in any workplace, organisation, institution or industry, but particularly in healthcare. In addition, it outlines how leaders can develop their leadership potential or see leadership from a new perspective. Research evidence for the theory of Congruent Leadership is introduced and the chapter concludes by exploring examples of congruent leaders.

CHAPTER 3: ATTRIBUTES OF CONGRUENT LEADERS

This chapter outlines the attributes and characteristics of congruent leaders. In doing so the chapter clarifies the parameters for understanding how to recognise a congruent leader. Other examples of congruent leaders are described at the conclusion to this chapter.

CHAPTER 4: VISION VERSUS VALUES

This chapter explores the difference in leadership theories when they are driven by two different primary areas of focus: vision and values. In the case of transformational leadership, the primary driver is the leader's vision. With Congruent Leadership the primary driver is the leader's values. This chapter will outline why this shift in focus matters if a values-based focus on leadership is to be understood and how a clear insight into this shift impacts upon grasping a values-based leadership theory such as Congruent Leadership. This chapter is supported by exploring examples of how congruent leaders have their values on show.

CHAPTER 5: THE STRENGTHS AND LIMITATIONS OF CONGRUENT LEADERSHIP

This chapter outlines the strengths and the limitations of Congruent Leadership theory. Congruent Leadership theory can only be that: a theory, until it is proven conclusively. This chapter suggests that Congruent Leadership theory is based on sound research design, data analysis, methodologies and a number of different studies, conducted over time, in different countries and with different professional groups. This chapter outlines arguments in support of, and against, the theory of Congruent Leadership. As with the previous chapters, this chapter concludes by offering further examples of congruent leaders.

THE CONTEXT OF CONGRUENT LEADERSHIP

CHAPTER 6: THE POWER OF SELF

This chapter outlines why knowing our values begins with knowing ourselves – what is important to us, what our aspirations are, how we relate to or interact with others and mostly how well we know who we are and what matters as we pass through life. This chapter explores what values are and offers strategies that may be useful in terms of helping us understand who we are, what we value and how these impact on our relationships with others. Fundamentally this chapter explores the relationship of 'self' in establishing effective Congruent Leadership with a number of other examples of congruent leaders provided to support this chapter.

CHAPTER 7: ORGANISATIONAL CULTURE AND CONGRUENT LEADERSHIP

This chapter addresses the relationship between organisational culture and leadership and the vital place Congruent Leadership can play in helping leaders shape or influence an organisation's culture. Congruent leaders are firmly focused on putting into practice their values, and as values are an open expression of culture there is a direct link between the activity of congruent leaders and their influence and impact on an organisation's culture (or indeed any area where a culture is evident). The chapter concludes by describing and exploring further examples of congruent leaders.

CHAPTER 8: THE APPLICATION OF CONGRUENT LEADERSHIP IN THE WORKPLACE

This chapter considers the way organisations and individuals can apply Congruent Leadership to enhance their leadership potential and bring about positive change in their workplace and professional lives. Practical approaches for health professionals from a range of practice disciplines are offered so that Congruent Leadership can be applied in the practice and healthcare domain. This chapter concludes by providing further examples of congruent leaders.

CHAPTER 9: SUMMARY: THE CONGRUENT LEADER

This chapter offers a summary of the theory of Congruent Leadership and suggests other examples of how this new approach to leadership can be understood as a valid theory for describing a way of applying and implementing values-based leadership.

ACKNOWLEDGEMENTS

No book is completely written by one person. The inspiration, ideas and support in many cases come from others. This book is no different. The inspirations, to a large extent, come from recognising that much of what is out there in text and educational institutions about leadership needs to be rethought, or at least conceptualised differently. Recognising that leaders are or can be anyone at any level or in any position needs to be reinforced and it was evident to me that few leadership theories shone a light on how this could be achieved. The ideas came from analysing the data and words of the many people who have taken part in the research projects that underpin this book. Without their participation, the new leadership theory (Congruent Leadership) explained in the book would not have been developed. In addition, I have many people to thank for their support. First and foremost is my wife Karen, who has read and reread transcript after transcript and listened to hours of dialogue as I outlined the theory and discussed the people I thought of as congruent leaders. A work colleague, Becky Broomfield, proofread the initial draft and offered sound and useful advice in the lead up to the final manuscript. Finally, I need to acknowledge the wonderful contribution of SAGE Publishing for agreeing to partner with me in seeing the book through to completion, particularly Donna Goddard for taking the project up on my behalf with SAGE. Also, dear reader, thank you for picking up this book and taking time to consider a new way to think about and practise values-based leadership.

PUBLISHER'S ACKNOWLEDGEMENTS

The publishers are grateful to the following academics for their constructive and critical feedback on the proposal for the book and subsequent draft material:

- Hazel Cowls, University of Plymouth
- Frank Donnelly, University of Adelaide
- Peter Ellis, Independent
- Adam Layland, Coventry University
- Claire Peers, University of Plymouth
- Zoe Wilkes, University of Hull
- Sue Gledhill, Australia Catholic University

LEADERSHIP BACKGROUND

1

LEADERSHIP: WHAT WE KNOW NOW

'Leadership is practiced not so much in words as in attitude and in actions.'

Harold Geneen, CEO of ITT, *Managing* (1984)

INTRODUCTION

This book proposes a new way to understand and describe leadership within the healthcare domain as well as in the wider world. As such, this chapter starts by outlining what might already be known about leadership and leadership theories, and to do so thoroughly we will explore theories from across the academic spectrum, a theme that will continue throughout the book.

Understanding leadership is not a new phenomenon. It has been a feature of military and political agendas for many centuries. However, it is only in the last century or so that an understanding of leadership has become of interest to educational, business, industry and medical or health service organisations. This has occurred as the pace of change in industry and society has increased and the need to deal with people in more inclusive and collaborative ways has been recognised as vital for industrial and societal success. In my professional life, very little was mentioned of leadership (beyond discussions of management) until the 1990s and it was only then that my interest was sparked. There are a plethora of books, journal articles, web pages and papers that elaborate upon a wide variety of theories, definitions and perspectives about how to recognise effective leadership, develop better leaders, promote change or innovation and promote more effective organisations. While the origins of the theory presented in this book are from the health domain, this chapter will draw on concepts, definitions and theories of leadership from a far wider circle of literature including business, industry, educational and the military. This chapter aims to clarify what leadership means and explore how it may be understood.

Gaining an insight into leadership is fraught with obstacles and the concept of leadership can be a tricky one to capture. This partly explains why so much has been written about it from so many different perspectives and, surprisingly, why it remains generally understood so superficially. Commonly it has been linked to theories of management and associated with elevated hierarchical positions and power. This book is not specifically directed at leaders of this ilk, e.g. people in authority, managers or senior managers. However, there is a great deal this book will offer these leaders too. Indeed, leadership and leaders are considered to be different from management and managers (Zaleznik, 1977; Kotter, 1990; Stanley, 2006, 2011, 2017) and it is acknowledged that management and leadership functions and attributes are related to each other. For the purposes of this book, concepts of management are not explicitly explored or considered. This is a book about leadership, and it is for anyone who could be described as or aspire to become a leader.

LEADERSHIP DEFINED

Many people from a range of different groups have been interested in discovering more about leadership and for a long time the nature of leadership has been extensively considered and researched (Swanwick and McKimm, 2011). Chinese and Indian scholars have studied and written about leadership for centuries. It is referred to in the Old Testament and numerous mythical stories from civilisations across the globe address the act of leadership. The famous Chinese scholar Confucius wrote about leadership, and Plato, who lived between 427 and 347 BCE, wrote *The Republic* about the value of developing leadership characteristics by describing the attributes required to navigate and command at sea (Adair, 2002a). In almost any field or endeavour, from leading large corporations and massive armies, to leading the parents committee of a local school, in the hospital ward or office football team, leadership and the experience of being a leader is a common theme.

Definitions of leadership are everywhere. Stogdill (1974, p. 7) believes that 'there are almost as many different definitions of leadership as there are people who have attempted to define the concept'. Northouse (2016, p. 2) too, indicates that as soon as 'we try to define leadership, we immediately discover that leadership has many different meanings'. Research by Bennis and Nanus (1985, p. 4) had them suggest that in relation to leadership, 'never have so many laboured so long to say so little'. I am almost apologetic for adding to the discussion. However, add to it I will although I hope to try and clarify leadership definitions and theories as we explore each of the theories. Understanding leadership in general is central to understanding the explanation of Congruent Leadership that follows and as such it is useful to begin with an exploration of the terms 'leadership' and 'leader'.

There is a wide variety of definitions, beliefs and perspectives on the topic of leadership with Fiedler (1967), who primarily studied military and managerial leadership, suggesting that the leader has long been considered to be the individual in the group with the task of coordinating and directing the group's activities. In the past, others have viewed leadership from a personality perspective, a power relationship perspective, as an instrument of goal achievement (Bass, 1990) or as part of a process of influencing people to accomplish goals (Northouse, 2016; Grossman and Valiga, 2013).

Leadership can also be viewed as achieving things with the support of others (Leigh and Maynard, 1995), and Wedderburn-Tate (1999, p. 107), writing from a healthcare perspective, feels that the leader's function is to get others to 'perform at consistently high levels, voluntarily'. This is in keeping with President Eisenhower's view that leadership is the art of getting someone else to do something you want done because they want to do it (Stanton et al., 2010, p. 3). These definitions suggest that influence is an accepted factor in leadership.

Fiedler (1967) and Dublin (1968) suggest leadership addresses more than an influence and propose that leadership is the exercise of authority and the making of decisions. They see the leader as the person who has formal authority (power) and functional capacity over a group. Maxwell (2002), however, supporting Leigh and Maynard (1995) and Wedderburn-Tate (1999), feels this is going too far and that leadership is influence, nothing more, nothing less. Stogdill (1950), writing from the insights of his seminal work, also feels that leadership and influence are related, although he believes it may also be more than just this. He proposes another view, that leadership is the process of influencing people or the activities of a group to accomplish goals (Stogdill, 1950). This perspective supports the concept of influence and acknowledges that people without formal power can exercise leadership. Leadership is also seen as 'a talent that each of us has and that can be learned, developed and nurtured. Most importantly it is not necessarily tied to a position of authority in an organisation' (Grossman and Valiga, 2013, p. 18).

As well as goal-setting and influence, Stogdill (1950) suggests that leadership is also an important element in effecting change. Kotter (1990, p. 40), writing much later, supports this, indicating that 'leadership is all about coping with change'. Bennis and Nanus (1985, p. 3) also understood that a leader is 'one who commits people to action, who converts followers into leaders and who converts leaders into agents of change'. In addition, Lipman (1964, p. 122), defines leadership from a business/management perspective as 'the initiation of a new structure or procedure for accomplishing an organisation's goals and objectives'.

These views appear to suggest that change is central to leadership and they rest on the assumption that leaders function within an organisation where change, rather than stability, is the goal. Pedler et al. (2004), also writing from a management perspective, indicates that leadership – while including elements of the leader's character and the context within which the leadership takes place – focuses on the critical tasks the leader must perform and the problems and challenges that leaders face, again, defining leadership by the leader's ability to change or respond to challenges.

Leadership has been viewed as attending to the meanings and values of the group rather than just the authority, function, challenges and traits of the leader. Covey (1992) described what he called 'principle-centred leadership' and Pondy (1978) similarly proposed that the ability to make activities meaningful and not necessarily to change behaviour – but to give others a sense of understanding of what they are doing – is at the core of leadership. These perspectives fall close to those proposed around Congruent Leadership. Covey (1992) and Pondy (1978) suggest that the act of leading is about making the meaning of an activity explicit. 'Unlike the supposed individualistic leadership of the past, now leadership is influenced by the impact of the immediate and surrounding context ... the contention put forward is that (the) organisational context(s) provides the parameters within which current leadership is contained' (Kakabadse and Kakabadse, 1999, p. 2). From this perspective it can be argued that the task of the leader is to interpret and clarify the context and thus provide a platform for communicating meaning within the activity.

As a result, leadership becomes more about selecting, synthesising and articulating an appropriate vision for the follower (Bennis et al., 1995). Greenfield (1986) also explored the concept of vision by suggesting that, rather than just clarifying the meaning or making the activity meaningful, leadership is about setting the meaning, describing leadership as 'a wilful act where one person attempts to construct the social world for others ... leaders will try to commit others to the values that they themselves believe are good and that organisations are built on the unification of people around values' (Greenfield, 1986, p. 166). Bell and Ritchie (1999) and Day et al. (2000), like Greenfield (1986), writing from an education perspective, commonly refer to the 'head teacher' as the person within a school who is responsible for 'establishing core characteristics' (Bell and Ritchie, 1999, p. 24) and for committing others to their values and setting the overall aims for the school.

However, no one definition can be considered wholly right or wrong and there are a multitude of other perspectives that have not been outlined above. There is considerable overlap and blurring at the edges too and these varied perspectives and definitions, while offering an eclectic view of leadership, may sit more comfortably alongside Duke's (1986, p. 10) suggestion that 'leadership seems to be a Gestalt phenomenon, greater than the sum of its parts.'

Therefore it is evident that leadership has been studied in many fields of endeavour, by many scholars and individuals for a very long time. However, rather than resulting in a clear and unequivocal understanding of leadership, many different and sometimes opposing definitions have evolved and exist (Swanwick and McKimm, 2011; Jones and Bennett, 2012; Rigolosi, 2013). These varied definitions could easily lead to confusion or unsettle the concept of leadership. Instead, I feel these definitions function like the dishes at a banquet, with each individual dish adding to the glory of the collective whole and each dish offering something that helps explain what leadership is and how leadership can be understood.

However, definitions alone offer only a taste of the meaning of leadership. A wider view may be more helpful. To this end, the next section explores the theoretical perspectives of leadership and brings a greater array of dishes to the banquet.

THEORIES AND STYLES

In order to further clarify information about leadership and leaders, it is prudent to explore the theories and concepts of leadership that are prominent in the literature. The theories and styles of leadership are not proposed in a linear way, although the later theories have grown from, or are at least a reaction to, earlier theories. The following pages offer only an introduction to leadership theories, but it is hoped they set the stage for a consideration of Congruent Leadership theory and an understanding of leadership in the wider context of this book.

THE GREAT MAN THEORY: BORN TO LEAD

The 'Great Man Theory' (Galton, 1869, cited in Morrison, 1993) is one of the earliest theories of leadership. It suggests that leadership is a matter of birth, with the characteristics of leadership being inherited or, as Man (2010) suggests, assigned by divine decree. Bennis and Nanus (1985, p. 5) explained this theory by saying 'those of the right breed could lead; all others must be led.' This theory is about individuals born into 'great' families being considered to be infused with the skills and characteristics of a leader. The Great Man Theory is the seat of a very old view of leadership, where monarchist ideals and a belief in the line of succession dominate.

THE BIG BANG THEORY: GREAT EVENTS MAKE GREAT LEADERS

The 'Big Bang Theory' proposed that calamitous circumstances provided the elements essential for the creation of leaders. Leaders, it suggests, were created by the great events that affected their lives (Grossman and Valiga, 2013). Here, the revolutions of the nineteenth and twentieth centuries and First World War are cited as examples of major calamitous circumstances, but this type of event could as easily be international or local terror events, such as the Lindt coffee shop siege in Sydney, or the Paris and London terror atrocities, or a natural disaster such as the Australian floods in 2011 and the Victorian fires in 2009 and 2015. The calamitous event could as easily be a family crisis or a personal catastrophe, such as the one that befell Malala Yousafzai in Pakistan and thrust leadership responsibilities onto her (see Chapter 7). Bennis and Nanus (1985, p. 5) explain this theory by saying that 'great events made leaders of otherwise ordinary people.' This suggests that it was the situation and the followers that combined to create the leader.

The lives of a number of great political and military leaders might be used to substantiate this theory of leadership. The life and rise to power of Napoleon Bonaparte following the after-effects of the French Revolution or the activism of Lech Walesa after martial law was imposed in Poland in the 1970s offer two examples of this theory in practice. The theory that otherwise ordinary people become great leaders because of great events may be true for some leaders but, as with Bonaparte or Walesa, much of this leader's success may be attributable to their hard work, courage and knowledge in preparation for the great events that unfold in their lifetime.

TRAIT THEORY: ATTRIBUTES ARE ALL

Another theory is the 'Trait Theory' of leadership. This theory rests on the assumption that the individual is more important than the situation. Thus it was proposed that the identification of distinguishing characteristics of successful leaders would give clues about leadership (Swanwick and McKimm, 2011; Grossman and Valiga, 2013). Rafferty (1993) and Jones and Bennett (2012) refer to this as the constitutional approach, where part of the assumption is that if great leaders cannot be trained or taught, they can at least be selected, linking this with attributes of the Great Man Theory.

A large number of studies in the early part of the twentieth century (Stogdill, 1948, 1974; Yoder-Wise, 2015; Mann, 1959; Kirkpatrick and Locke, 1991; Smith, 1999; Grossman and Valiga, 2013; Northouse, 2016) were initiated to consider the traits of the great leaders. However, as Bass (1990) indicates, while a number of traits did seem to correspond with leadership, no qualities were found that were universal to all leaders. Stogdill (1948), who undertook a major review of universal leadership traits between 1904 and 1947, concluded that no consistent set of traits differentiated leaders from non-leaders in a range of work environments and situations. The traits Stogdill identified in 1948 and again in 1974, and others identified by Mann (1959), Kirkpatrick and Locke (1991), Smith (1999) and Grossman and Valiga (2013), are listed in Table 1.1.

The descriptive words on these lists indicate that trait theories have evolved and changed with time, but all remain unable to capture any great degree of consistency between the traits identified. Stogdill found in 1948 and again in 1974 that the traits that lead to success may differ according to the situation the leader is in, as well as the personality of the leader. Therefore the traits themselves could be seen as misleading, although it was suggested that the leader's characteristics play a critical part in effective leadership (Northouse, 2016). It is also suggested that possession of all of the traits is an impossible ideal and there is a considerable number of cases where people who possess a few, or even none, of the principal traits achieve notable success as leaders (Stogdill, 1974).

Table 1.1 Leadership traits

Stogdill, 1948 (cited in Northouse, 2016, p. 18)		Mann (1959, p. 253)	
Intelligence	Alertness	Intelligence	Masculinity
Insight	Responsibility	Adjustment	Dominance
Initiative	Persistence	Extroversion	Conservatism
Self-control	Sociability		

Stogdill, 1974 (cited in Northouse, 2016, p. 18)		Kirkpatrick and Locke (1991, p. 52)	
Achievement	Persistence	Drive	Motivation
Insight	Initiative	Integrity	Confidence
Self-confidence	Responsibility	Cognitive ability	Task knowledge
Cooperativeness	Tolerance		
Influence	Sociability		

Smith (1999, p. 6)	Grossman and Valiga (2013, p. 5)
Early loss of a parent	Abundant reserves of energy
Escape from squalor (coming from a socially disadvantaged position)	Ability to maintain a high level of activity
First-born child	A better education
Tall	Superior judgement
High energy levels	Decisiveness
Work long hours	Breadth of general knowledge
Can manage with little sleep	High degree of verbal facility
Introverted and psychologically on edge	Good interpersonal skills
Outsiders coming from beyond the group they lead	Self-confidence
Enormous self-belief	Creativity
	Above average height and weight

The disadvantage of Trait Theory is that it does not lead to a comprehensive theory of leadership and it neglects both the impact of the situational context within which the leader operates (Stogdill, 1948; Northouse, 2016), as well as the impact of the leader's personality (Mann, 1959). Rafferty (1993) also points out that trait theory ignores or underestimates the degree to which the leader's role could be structured by issues of class, gender or racial inequalities and it assumes a passive role for the followers.

Trait Theory developed as an elaboration of the Great Man Theory and remains central to what Grint (2000) described as 'the arts of leadership'. However, the investigation and establishment of Trait Theory developed in line with business and management development in the early twentieth century (Northouse, 2016), where it was hoped that once the appropriate qualities and traits were identified, a potential leader could be hired who demonstrated these traits, or a leader could be supported to acquire them through study and experience (Bernhard and Walsh, 1990). Then, if the appropriate conditions prevailed or could be predicted, appropriate people (who showed the relevant traits) could be selected or trained for the leadership situation. While it is possible to acquire some (but not all) of the traits, this theory remains divorced from the notion that leadership (in isolation from the traits) could be learnt and, as such, it found limited purchase with the liberated and increasingly educated masses of the

Western world. Therefore, as community values altered and research about leadership increased, other perspectives of leadership developed (Lett, 2002).

STYLE THEORY: IT'S ABOUT THE LEADER'S BEHAVIOUR

Another view of leadership can be seen by considering 'Style Theories' of leadership (Swanwick and McKimm, 2011). Studies of leadership and management and their relationship to productivity and group behaviour resulted in what are generally called Style Theories (Handy, 1999; Adair, 1998; Northouse, 2016). Style Theories explore how leaders behave, what they do, how they act, as well as how groups respond, with leaders being described as either democratic, paternalistic, laissez-faire, authoritarian and/or dictatorial (Handy, 1999; Lett, 2002; Northouse, 2016) (see Table 1.2). As these words were found to have an 'emotive connotation', aspects of Style Theory are also described as 'structuring and supportive styles' (Handy, 1999 p. 101), and much of the literature related to Style Theory emphasises the benefits or drawbacks of one or another approach to motivating a group (usually of subordinates to the leader).

Table 1.2   Management/leadership styles

Autocratic: characterised by being highly directive, viewed as having a right to manage.	
Positive points: clear objective, single-minded, based on orders, no thinking required.	**Negative points:** diminished autonomy, problem if the vision is false or off, power vacuum if the leader leaves, no debate, no opportunity to experience power before promotion.
Paternalistic: characterised by a caring but overprotective, interfering manager. Manager knows best, may consult, but the manager always decides. High degree of support but no corresponding responsibility or autonomy.	
Positive points: followers/employees may feel 'cared for', may foster a sense that they belong or have a team or esprit de corps.	**Negative points:** stifles autonomy. High reliance on the manager/organisation, even for basic human needs (like some 1970s Japanese companies: when some employees were off sick they felt so lost without their work they were encouraged to come in and spend their time, even if ill, with their colleagues and co-workers).
Democratic: characterised by discussion, debate and shared vision.	
Positive points: promotes a shared vision, ownership of outcomes and problems, involvement of the whole team, flatter structure employed.	**Negative points:** can allow the more vocal or more outspoken to dominate; mob may rule and may be wrong. Can lead to ineffective decision-making.
Laissez faire: characterised by an easy-going, non-directive and non-hierarchical approach.	
Positive points: promotes autonomy, self-survival, self-direction, individuality, freedom and self-expression.	**Negative points:** assumes everyone is willing or capable of leadership, or that people are happy to be left to their own devices. This approach can lead to chaos or anarchy.

Early investigations of Style Theory were undertaken by the Ohio State University in the 1960s, where a Leader Behaviour Description Questionnaire (LBDQ) was developed and tested in educational, military and industrial settings. Leaders, they concluded, exhibited either *structuring* behaviour that defined the work context and role responsibilities of subordinates, or *consideration* behaviours that focused on building relationships such as trust and respect with subordinates. These studies were elaborated on by the University of Michigan with an approach more focused on the leader's behaviours in relation to the performance of small groups (Northouse, 2016).

By the late 1960s Blake and Mouton (1964) had developed the 'Managerial Grid' (now called the 'Leadership Grid') as a model to support organisational leadership and management training, by exploring how leaders (managers) could help organisations reach their potential through either developing support for production or concern for people. The Management/Leadership Grid (Blake and Mouton, 1964; Blake and McCanse, 1991) can be used to explain how leaders or managers within an organisation function by focusing on the relationship between two factors. The first, *concern for people*, deals with how a manager or leader supports people within an organisation as they try to work towards their goals (Blake and Mouton, 1964). The other factor, *concern for results*, addresses how the manager/leader achieves various tasks and can include aspects such as policies, sales figures, quality targets and other activities and processes concerned with production or the organisation's goals. The Management/Leadership Grid is used to explain the Style Theory approach to leadership; however, it is not designed to instruct leaders in how to behave, but it is useful in supporting leaders (managers) in identifying the major components of their behaviour. The Style Theory, however, failed to elaborate on why some leaders were successful in certain situations and not in others (see Table 1.2).

Different organisations require different styles of management or leadership at different times, depending on their approach, goals and the stage of the organisation's development. Many authors use different terms (democratic = participative) but often they end up describing the same thing. It was Kurt Lewin who in 1948 set out the three basic leadership/management styles of autocratic, democratic and laissez-faire. Since then, other terms have been used and other views expressed. Here are some others:

- *Supporting:* Leaders pass day-to-day decisions to the followers. Leaders facilitate, influence and take part in decisions, but control is with the followers.
- *Delegating:* Leaders are still involved in decision-making and problem-solving but control is with the followers. While leaders may still retain some influence, the followers decide when and how the leaders will be involved.
- *Directing:* Leaders define the roles and tasks of the followers and supervise them closely. Decisions are made by the leader and announced, so communication is largely one-way.
- *Coaching:* Leaders still define roles and tasks but seek ideas and suggestions from the followers. Decisions remain the leader's prerogative, but communication is much more two-way.

Leaders also provide influence or/and resources to facilitate each of the types of styles outlined so that leaders are also seen as enablers, facilitators and guides in support of these approaches. There are a number of other views on the various styles of leadership. The style that individuals use will be based on a combination of their beliefs, values and preferences, as well as the organisational culture and norms which encourage some styles and discourage others. Examples are:

- charismatic leadership;
- participatory leadership;
- situational leadership;
- transactional leadership;
- transformational leadership;
- the quiet leader.

Clearly, some of these relate to specific leadership theories and this is where the matter of styles and theories becomes intertwined. Tannenbaum and Schmidt (1958) suggest there are seven leadership styles, Tayeb (1996) suggests there are four and Morgan (1986) proposes six styles of leadership (and management). Confused yet? I'd be surprised if you weren't. Goleman et al. (2002) suggest that there are six styles: coaching, visionary, affiliative, democratic, pace-setting and commanding, although as you will see from any random internet search (with 'leadership styles' as the search phrase), there are many more.

SITUATIONAL OR CONTINGENCY THEORY: NO ONE BEST WAY

To address the failure of Style Theory and to elaborate on why some leaders are successful in certain situations and not in others, Fiedler (1967) proposed the 'Situational' or 'Contingency Theory' of leadership (Wedderburn-Tate, 1999) that was popularised by Hersey and Blanchard in 1982 (Swanwick and McKimm, 2011). Here, Fiedler (1967) and others (Tannenbaum and Schmit, 1958; Vroom and Yetton, 1973; House and Mitchell, 1974; Hersey and Blanchard, 1982) believed that leadership effectiveness was dependent on the relationship between the leader's task at hand, the leader's interpersonal skills and the favourableness of the work situation. Fiedler (1967) found after what has more recently been criticised as limited research (Handy, 1999) that leaders were more effective if the situation they were trying to function within was more favourable to them or, surprisingly, less favourable. The three factors relate to:

- the degree of trust and respect that the followers have for the leader;
- the clarity of the objectives to be achieved; and
- the degree of power in terms of whether the leader could reward or punish the followers or if the leader had clear organisational backing.

(Handy, 1999, pp. 103–5)

From Fiedler's perspective the key to understanding leadership is to be able to adapt the leadership approach to complement the issue being faced or to determine the appropriate action based on the people involved and the prevailing situation (Adair, 1998). Adair (1998) also offers an example of how situational leadership might be applied by describing the actions of a group of survivors following a shipwreck:

> The soldier in the party might take command if natives attacked them, the builder might organize the work of erecting houses and the farmer might direct the labour of growing food ... leadership would pass from member to member according to the situation. (Adair, 1998, p. 15)

Central to Fiedler's (1967) work was the ability to analyse how the leader could use power and influence without losing respect and credibility within the subordinate group. Tannenbaum and Schmit (1958) felt that organisations could help more by either structuring the task, improving the formal power of the leader or changing the composition of the follower group to give the leader a more favourable climate to work in. Criticism of Fiedler's situational–contingency model is that leadership is broader than the extent of the relationship between the three central factors while Handy (1999) also feels that this theory is not complicated enough to fully describe and address the convoluted nature of leadership.

Blanchard et al. (1994, p. 8) suggest that situational leadership is best used to support the activity of management and as a 'practical approach to managing and motivating people'. They add that it has been 'taught to managers at all levels of most of the Fortune 500 companies as well as to managers in fast-growing entrepreneurial organisations'. As a result, the distinction between theories of leadership and management remained closely intertwined and although Zaleznik (1977) and Kotter (1990) make it clear that management and leadership are different, many of the perspectives and theories that developed to explore and explain leadership have grown from a desire to understand human resource management, improve employee and workforce production and support the development of managers.

TRANSFORMATIONAL LEADERSHIP THEORY: CHANGE IS THE FOCUS

In an attempt to understand the distinction between leadership and management and to address the question of why some leaders are able to inspire their followers even when the situation is less than ideal the theory of 'Transformational Leadership' was developed (Northouse, 2016). The term was coined by Downton (1973) and later adopted and developed by House (1976) and Burns (1978), who really secured the term's distinction by firmly linking the leaders' and the followers' motives. It was Bass (1985) though, while seeking to identify the distinctions between leadership and management, who later refined the theory and felt that

Transformational Leadership motivated the followers to do more than was expected by providing an idealised influence, inspirational motivation and vision. Transformational Leadership is also strongly associated with the qualitative studies of Bennis and Nanus (1985) and, more recently, Fuda (2014). These scholars also sought to tease out the distinction between management and leadership, with Transformational Leadership seen as connected to a process of attending to the needs of the followers, so that the interaction of each raised the motivation and energy of the other. Kakabadse and Kakabadse (1999) and Swanwick and McKimm (2011) suggest that Transformational Leadership is about challenging the status quo, creating a vision and sharing that vision, with successful transformational leaders being able to establish and gain support for their vision while being consistently and persistently driven towards maintaining momentum and empowering others.

Bennis and Nanus (1985), in expanding on Burns' (1978) theory, identified four themes that they felt were pivotal to effective Transformational Leadership:

- *vision* – the ability to have a dream and to actually deliver on it;
- *communication* – the ability to articulate the vision so that it steals into the imagination and the minds of the followers;
- *trust* – the ability of the followers to feel that their leader is consistent, has integrity and can be relied on;
- *self-knowledge (self-knowing)* – which Bennis and Nanus (1985, p. 57) described as the ability to 'know their worth and trust themselves without letting their ego or image get in the way'.

In effect, 'self-knowing' is about looking for the fit between who they (the leaders) are and who they need to be to fulfil the task. Handy (1999, p. 117) aligned 'self-knowing' with 'emotional wisdom'. While Goleman (1996) and Goleman et al. (2002) have elaborated on this aspect of leadership, connecting it to the concept of 'emotional intelligence' where a person is able to motivate themselves, be creative and perform at their peak, sensing what others are feeling and handling relationships effectively. The transformational leader need not be associated with status or power and is seen as being appropriate at all levels of an organisation. In effect, their role is in communicating a vision that gives meaning to the work of others and, crucially, the role of the transformational leader is in the reconstruction of the context in which people work, removing the old and replacing it with the new.

The interdependence of followers and leaders within this theory has meant that Transformational Leadership has found favour in a number of fields, such as education and healthcare (Day et al., 2000; Welford, 2002; Thyer, 2003; Goertz Koerner, 2010; Freshwater et al., 2009; Weberg, 2010; Marshall, 2011; Swanwick and McKimm, 2011; Casida and Parker, 2011; Hutchinson and Jackson, 2012; Jones and Bennett, 2012; Tinkham, 2013; Ross et al., 2014; Lavoie-Tremblay et al., 2015; Weng et al., 2015). It is also suggested that Transformational Leadership is a suitable leadership approach for empowering followers and supporting them within an organisation.

The NHS Confederation (1999) indicated that, in their view, Transformational Leadership is best suited to the modern leadership of the NHS. In addition, Weng et al. (2015) suggest, in a substantial Taiwanese research study, that there is a significant correlation between Transformational Leadership and innovation within the health arena. Casida and Parker (2011), in a study in the USA, likewise suggested that leaders who demonstrated a transformational style were seen to be making an extra effort, achieving greater satisfaction and being more effective, while Lavoie-Tremblay et al. (2015) suggested that supportive leadership practices were able to impact upon increasing retention and improving productivity.

Transformational Leadership has gained favour because it is related to the establishment of a vision and adapting to change. However, Hutchinson and Jackson (2012) state there is limited robust critical review or empirical exploration of this theory and how it may apply in some work fields. Rafferty (1993, p. 8) warns that the 'charismatic' element of Transformational Leadership can be 'potentially exploitative' if the leader takes advantage of conflict in the needs or values system of the followers. However, it is in this area of potential weakness that Kakabadse and Kakabadse (1999) see the power of Transformational Leadership, indicating that it offers the leader the opportunity to penetrate the soul and psyche of others and increases the level of awareness that motivates people to strive for greater ends.

TRANSACTIONAL LEADERSHIP THEORY: LEADER AS MANAGER

Burns (1978) describes 'Transactional Leadership' as the antithesis of 'Transformational Leadership', indicating that transactional leadership exists where there is an exchange relationship between the leader and the followers (Jones and Bennett, 2012). Here, the role of the transactional leader is to focus on the purpose of the organisation and to assist people to recognise what needs to be done in order to reach a desired outcome. A reward/punishment feedback process is used as a motivator (Jones and Bennett, 2012), with Kakabadse and Kakabadse (1999) describing transactional leadership as the skill and ability required to deal with the mundane, operational and day-to-day transactions of organisational life. The transactional leader keeps meetings on track, keeps to the agenda and conducts appraisals on subordinates (Kakabadse and Kakabadse, 1999). Transactional Leadership is also known as 'Transactional Management' with transactional leaders used to keep order, effectively manage the more routine tasks and retain their credibility by keeping the staff on track to meet the organisation's goals (Burns, 1978).

Criticism of this leadership theory is that it relies on procedures, technicality and hard data to inform decision-making, with Day et al. (2000, p. 4) describing it as a form of 'Scientific Managerialism' that relies on the assumption that leaders are in a position to control rewards. It is also criticised by Rafferty (1993) because it relies on the belief that human behaviour is driven by motivation for reward and an incentive system. Rafferty (1993, p. 8) also criticises transactional leadership because it is prone to being 'more conservative than creative'. The rationale behind transactional leadership is that in order for leaders to function effectively they should be able to control the context within which they are required to lead, in effect managing their environment and limiting change.

AUTHENTIC THEORY/BREAKTHROUGH LEADERSHIP: TRUE TO YOUR VALUES

'Authentic Leadership' (Bhindi and Duignan, 1997; George, 2003; Avolio and Gardner, 2005; Cantwell, 2015) and 'Breakthrough Leadership' (Sarros and Butchatsky, 1996) are more recent leadership theories. Both of these perspectives of leadership point towards an approach where leaders are thought to be true to their own values and beliefs, and the leader's credibility rests on their integrity and ability to be seen as a role model because of these values and beliefs. The 'Breakthrough' leader and 'Authentic' leader respect and listen to others and are guided by their passion and meaning, purpose and values (Sarros and Butchatsky, 1996; Bhindi and Duignan 1997; George, 2003; Avolio and Gardner, 2005; Cantwell, 2015). Cantwell (2015, p. 33), in his excellent book *Leadership in Action*, when discussing Authentic Leadership, goes as far as suggesting that Authentic Leadership is the foundation of leadership, and that 'values determined the authenticity of a leader'.

In 2005, the American Association of Critical-Care Nurses published a statement aimed at helping establish healthy work environments. The basis for this was a list of six 'standards' based on Authentic Leadership. They were described as:

- skilled communication;
- true collaboration;
- effective decision-making;
- appropriate staffing;
- meaningful recognition;
- authentic leadership.

As such, Authentic Leadership was described as the 'glue' used to hold a healthy work environment together (Shirley, 2006), with leaders being encouraged to engage with employees and promote positive behaviours. Wong and Cummings (2009), writing from a healthcare perspective, also suggest that Authentic Leadership was a suitable theory for aligning future leadership practice. Writers such as Gonzalez (2012) have taken Authentic Leadership further and describe what they call 'Mindful Leadership', where leaders employ self-awareness and self-leadership principles while being mindful of their impact on others. This theory sits most closely in alignment with Congruent Leadership.

SERVANT LEADERSHIP THEORY: A FOLLOWER TO LEAD

In keeping with some of the key elements of Authentic Leadership, 'Servant Leadership' focuses on the leader's stewardship role and encourages leaders to 'serve' others while staying in tune with the organisation's goals and values (Swanwick and McKimm, 2011; Jones and Bennett, 2012). The concept of Servant Leadership was coined and defined by Robert Greenleaf (1977), who stated that servant leaders rely less on hierarchical positions and more on collaboration, trust, empathy and the use of ethical power (see Box 1.1).

A number of authors have emphasised the relevance of Servant Leadership as a model to support organisations because of its focus on promoting user involvement and collaboration (Anderson, 2003; Kerfoot, 2004; Swearingen and Liberman, 2004; Campbell and Rudisill, 2005; Peete, 2005; Robinson, 2006; Thorne, 2006; Walker, 2006; Swanwick and McKimm, 2011; Jones and Bennett, 2012). It is also valued as a model to support staff or employees and influence retention (Swearingen and Liberman, 2004). Hanse et al. (2015, p. 5), in a significant Swedish study, were able to show that nurse managers who demonstrated Servant Leadership had stronger 'exchange relationships' in terms of 'empowerment', 'humility' and 'stewardship' with followers. Their results reinforced the notion that Servant Leadership was relevant and suited to service-orientated organisations with benefits for supporting, valuing and developing people.

BOX 1.1   TEN PRINCIPLES OF SERVANT LEADERSHIP

- Listening
- Conceptualisation
- Empathy
- Foresight
- Healing
- Stewardship
- Awareness
- Commitment to the growth of people
- Persuasion
- Building community

Servant Leadership is also valued because its key principles (Spears, 1995) (Box 1.1) support caring and compassion and these seem to fit appropriately within supportive organisational principles. Eicher-Catt (2005), however, believes Servant Leadership is a myth that is unworkable in the real world, and that it fails to live up to its promise of being gender-neutral. In fact, because of the paradoxical language and apposition of 'servant' and 'leader', this accentuates gender bias, so that it ends up supporting androcentric patriarchal norms (Eicher-Catt, 2005). There is also an argument put forward by Avolio and Gardener (2005) that Servant Leadership has not been developed from an empirical base and is therefore purely theoretical.

ACTIVITY 1.1   REFLECTIVE EXERCISE

Consider all of the theories outlined above and make a list that compares and contrasts the pros and cons for each. Some will be obvious, others quite subtle. Consider each theory and whether it will be useful to support your clinical/professional practice or enhance interprofessional collaboration.

CHAPTER SUMMARY

The essence of the Great Man, Trait and Style Theories of leadership is that the individual leader is critical but the context is not. Therefore as long as the right leader with the appropriate leadership qualities is found or selected, the leader will be able to lead under any circumstances. These theories imply that organisations, businesses, healthcare providers, the military and other groups should concern themselves with the search for and development of leaders rather than be preoccupied with the context within which they will have to operate. Indeed, this has been the approach taken by many organisations and much of the literature related to leadership from a military, political, religious and business basis revolved around describing the lives and achievements of highly regarded military generals, political juggernauts, religious figureheads and captains of industry (Fest, 1974; Grabsky, 1993; D'Este, 1996; Hibbert, 1998; Useem, 1998; Grint, 2000; Krause, 2000; Adair, 2002a; Mandela, 1994; Harvey, 1998; Danzig, 2000; Carwardine, 2003; Gallagher et al., 2003; Carson, 1999; Banks, 1982; Lacey, 1986; Clemmer and McNeil, 1989; Allan, 1992; Branson, 1998; Useem, 1998; Danzig, 2000; Kouzes and Posner, 2003).

The Situational or Contingency Theory, and to a small degree the Big Bang Theory of leadership, imply that both the individual and the context are fundamental. These theories describe the leader as being aware of their own leadership skills and of the context within which they lead, so that they can plan for the degree of alignment between their leadership approach and the situation they are in. For example, where a crisis occurs and a strong leader is available, this leader can step forward to lead and only step back (if required) when the situation changes and the context is no longer conducive to their vigorous approach. Leadership is arrived at by supporting the leader to be self-aware and by situational analysis so that, in effect, certain situations demand certain types of leader. Skilful leaders may be able to adapt their style to suit particular situations and, as such, the leader's behaviour or actions may change to suit the situation at hand. These theories of leadership found favour in, and developed from, research and literature derived from management and business perspectives (Blanchard et al., 1994; Adair, 1998; Adair, 2002b; Northouse, 2016); while transformational and transactional theories of leadership also developed as researchers sought to explore the differences between leadership and management (Bennis and Nanus, 1985; Bass, 1990).

If leadership is seen to be about unifying people around values, constructing a social world for others around those values and then helping people get through change, identifying a leadership theory that will facilitate people to understand the application of leadership in their organisational environment or situation is important. In this context, Authentic Leadership or Servant Leadership may be appropriate. However, they are not based on extensive empirical work and may not be as well developed as they need to be to effectively support the application of a values-based leadership approach.

To this end, the next chapter explores elements of leadership from the perspective of a new leadership theory: *Congruent Leadership*. This theory is based on significant empirical research specifically undertaken within the healthcare environment and with a wide range of health professionals over a number of years and in different counties. The new theory is offered as an alternative to older or other leadership theories by drawing upon a direct link between the values the leader holds and their actions.

CONGRUENT
LEADERSHIP
OUTLINED

2

CONGRUENT LEADERSHIP THEORY

We are what we think.

All that we are arises with our thoughts.

With our thoughts we make the world.

Speak or act with a pure mind

And happiness will follow you

As your shadow, unshakable.

The Dhammapada (from a collection of sayings from Buddha)

INTRODUCTION

This chapter will elaborate on Congruent Leadership theory, what it means, how it is defined and what it constitutes. This chapter also highlights how Congruent Leadership is related to power, quality processes, innovation and change, and why it offers a solid foundation for leaders in healthcare, or indeed any workplace, industry, institution, organisation or business. Research evidence is offered through-out the chapter to support the claim that Congruent Leadership theory can help healthcare professionals develop and achieve their leadership potential even if they are not in positions of seniority or management authority. The chapter concludes (as do many of the further chapters) by exploring examples of congruent leaders who display their values and beliefs and who lead by matching the values and beliefs with their actions.

CONGRUENT LEADERSHIP THEORY

Congruent Leadership can be defined as a match (congruence) between the leader's values and beliefs and their actions (Stanley, 2006a, 2006b, 2008, 2011, 2017). Leaders are identified as such because they are driven to act in ways consistent with their values and it is for this reason that they are seen as leaders and followed. Congruent leaders may have a vision and idea about where they want to go, but this is not why they are followed. Congruent Leadership is based on the leader's values, beliefs and principles and is about where the leader stands, not where they are going. This approach to leadership is paralleled by Kouzes and Posner's (2010, p. xxii) description of leadership where they suggest that 'values drive commitment', adding that 'people want to know what you stand for and believe in.' Congruent leaders are motivational, inspirational, organised, effective communicators and builders of relationships. They commonly have no formal, structured or hierarchical position in an organisation but they may have, and if they do, it is not their position that motivates their followers, but their values and beliefs as evidenced by their actions.

Congruent leaders appear to be guided by passion, compassion, commitment, courage and respect for others. It is these attributes that makes this theory particularly relevant for those working in service industries or the healthcare sector, although it can be applied and recognised in any workplace or organisation. Congruent leaders build enduring relationships with others, stand the test of their principles and are more concerned with supporting the empowerment of others than with power or their own prestige. Kouzes and Posner (2010, p. 34) support these principles suggesting that 'if you are ever to become a leader whom others willingly follow, you must be known as someone who stands by his or her principles.' This is true of leaders at all levels, but this theory may be of more value for leaders without formal authority or status. The research that underpins the development of this theory was undertaken in the health sector and it explains why and how nurses and other health professionals and many non-titled or non-hierarchically positioned leaders, or indeed leaders at all levels, could function and be effective without formal influence in the health service or in the wider health organisation.

THE RESEARCH BEHIND CONGRUENT LEADERSHIP

The theory of Congruent Leadership initially developed from the results of my doctoral research and a series of subsequent studies that have explored clinical leadership from the perspective of a number of health professional disciplines. The initial research was undertaken with registered nurses at a large acute hospital in the UK between 2001 and 2004. This was followed with five further research projects that explored the phenomenon of clinical leadership from the perspective of paramedics (in 2008), senior registered nurses and managers in the aged care arena (in 2012), ambulance volunteers (in 2013) and allied health professionals, mainly dietetics, occupational therapists, physiotherapists, social workers, podiatrists and speech therapists (between 2014 and 2015), in Australia and rural and remote nurses in Western NSW (Australia) in 2017. It was soon clear that none of the previously established leadership theories described or supported the results that began to emerge from the research. As such, a new leadership theory focused on values-based leadership was needed.

Congruent Leadership is proposed as a new theory to frame and understand leadership in the health service (although the theory can be extrapolated to other domains such as the military, business and education). It is proposed as a theory to better explain and understand leadership predominantly located in the clinical area, at the bedside, at the roadside and across all healthcare-related disciplines where a foundation of values is vital. Beyond this, Congruent Leadership can be used to explain some leadership approaches at the white/black board, at the actual coalface, on the battlefield and in the office or wider workplace. This section of the chapter sets out to explain the research evidence that supported the origins of Congruent Leadership.

IT ALL STARTED WITH CLINICAL LEADERSHIP

At the time I started to explore clinical leadership the dominant leadership theory supporting clinical and healthcare leadership was Transformational Leadership (Marriner-Tomey, 2009). However, Transformational Leadership theory is based on the leader's vision and how that vision is communicated to those who see them as leaders (or are told they are their leaders, e.g. managers). In the course of the research described below, having a vision or being visionary was seldom identified by respondents as being relevant or significant. Clinically focused leaders in the initial and subsequent research were rarely described as having or requiring the attribute of being visionary. This led to the conclusion that established leadership theories that rested on 'vision' as the basis for the leadership theory were unable to describe the type of leadership displayed by clinically focused leaders.

There were other theoretical perspectives to consider. Australian authors, Bhindi and Duignan (1997) described what they called 'Authentic Leadership' where in order to lead; leaders were required to be true to themselves, with this approach to leadership based on the leader's personal credibility and integrity. This was followed by George (2003) who also described 'Authentic Leadership' where leaders served others through their leadership and by focusing on their values. These views build upon Pondy's (1978) description of leadership, where leaders are encouraged to explore their values and lead from recognition of what was identified as important.

In the research studies described shortly, time and time again what stood out as important were values in action and respondents made comments that supported or pointed to the idea that clinically focused leaders, or those who were described as clinical leaders, were rarely seen to be driven by or heard to be articulating a vision. Respondents commonly said things like, 'that one' (as they pointed from the interview room when a particular person passed the door) 'That one, she is a clinical leader ... if my mother becomes sick, she's the one I'd want to look after her ... she cares.' Or they might say, 'I have been encouraged to move into management, but in my heart of hearts I know this is not for me. I came into nursing (or any other health discipline) to care for people and I want to stay focused on that.' Or I heard people describe their frustration if their values were being compromised by health service or management demands to (in their view) diminish client contact or divide their time away from principally caring activities.

It was evident that it was the leaders' *actions* based on *their values and beliefs* that drew people to identify them as clinical leaders. They were generally clinically competent, but it was more than this that supported their being seen as leaders. It was the synergy of values between the person identifying the leader and the leaders' actions that prompted them to be seen as leaders. Followers were seeking or identifying leaders because they were practising in accordance with their values and beliefs, and not simply articulating a vision for others to follow.

Six completed research studies have been undertaken that have led to and support the development of Congruent Leadership theory. They are offered in outline below.

STUDY 1   IN COMMAND OF CARE: CLINICAL NURSE LEADERSHIP

Aim: To identify who the clinical leaders are in a large NHS Trust in the English Midlands and to explore and critically analyse the experience of being a clinical nurse leader.

Location: Worcestershire Acute NHS Trust in the English Midlands, UK.

Dates: February 2001 – December 2004.

Methodology: Qualitative – grounded theory methods – Pilot study then questionnaire and interviews.

Target group: Registered/qualified nurses (D to H Grade) in 36 clinical areas (in three hospitals) across one NHS Acute Trust.

Analysis: Interviews = NVivo 0.6 and manual data configuration questionnaire = SPSS.

Sample: Interviews n = 50 (42 RNs/8 clinical leaders) questionnaires 850 sent out; 188 returned (22.6 per cent).

Gender mix: Questionnaire: Female = 95 per cent / Male = 5 per cent; Interviews: Female = 100 per cent / Male = 0 per cent.

Ethics: West Midlands South Strategic Health Authority: Hereford and Worcester Local Research Ethics Committee; LREC 02/43 and permission from Worcester Royal Hospital DON.

Results: Clinical leaders were recognised because they were approachable, clinically competent and visible in practice, made effective decisions and communicated well. They were seen to be empowered and positive clinical role models who, most importantly, displayed their values and beliefs and held fast to their guiding principles about care and nursing.

The attribute least likely to be associated with clinical leadership was 'controlling'. The data suggested that another leadership theory was needed to support clinically focused leadership. This was where Congruent Leadership was initiated. This grew from both the questionnaire and interview results that suggested that clinical leaders were followed because their colleagues and peers saw the leaders' actions as a translation of their values and beliefs into practice. Clinical leaders were evident in large numbers and represented a wide range of levels of staff, but most commonly it was the most senior clinically focused nurses and rarely the ward managers who were selected or identified as clinical leaders. As well, the clinical leaders seemed to be more commonly identified in specialist areas of practice, such as accident and emergency and intensive care areas (where more experienced nurses commonly worked). Clinical leaders were often unaware that they had followers and commonly clinical leaders were not 'tagged' to titled or senior positions. The common theme was that clinical leaders had their values on show and these were based on a foundation of care. As well, many of the clinical leaders suggested that they faced issues of role conflict and struggled to maintain their 'clinical focus' in the face of 'management demands'.

STUDY 2   PERCEPTIONS OF CLINICAL LEADERSHIP IN THE ST JOHN AMBULANCE SERVICE IN WESTERN AUSTRALIA

Aim: To identify how clinical leadership is perceived by paramedics and ambulance personnel in the course of their everyday work and the effectiveness and consequences of the application of clinical leadership in pre-hospital care delivery.

Location: Western Australia (metropolitan, rural and remote areas of practice).

Dates: February – November 2010.

(Continued)

(Continued)

Methodology: Qualitative – phenomenology method – questionnaire.

Target group: 250 paramedics (non-volunteer) and ambulance officers who attended in-service education between February and November 2010 in Perth Western Australia.

Analysis: Questionnaire = SPSS and spreadsheet.

Sample: 250 questionnaires distributed, 104 returned = 41.6 per cent return rate.

Gender mix: Questionnaires: Female = 36 per cent / Male = 64 per cent.

Ethics: Ethical approval was sought and secured through the Curtin University Human Research Ethics Committee (Nu: SON&M 1-2010).

Results: In relation to the characteristics of a clinical leader most suggested that clinical leaders needed to be clinically competent (96 per cent), be a role model for others (93 per cent), be an effective communicator (89 per cent), inspire confidence (85 per cent), be approachable (96 per cent), have integrity (93 per cent), be supportive (91 per cent), be a decision-maker (87 per cent), be visible in practice (86 per cent) and set direction (87 per cent). Just over 84 per cent indicated (in keeping with the previous study) that 'controlling' was the attribute least associated with clinical leadership. Under half saw themselves as clinical leaders, although over one-third felt they could not engage in leadership activities for a range of reasons, including a lack of encouragement, lack of training opportunities, work pressures and a lack of opportunity to be leaders. Almost 60 per cent indicated that they faced barriers to becoming or deploying clinical leadership, with many indicating that they faced resistance from colleagues, no opportunities, the current management culture and a lack of experience.

In terms of formal leadership training, only 40.6 per cent indicated that they had had some sort of formal leadership training (although it was not clear what this constituted). In terms of formal management training 26 per cent indicated that they had had some sort of management training. The gender make-up of the respondents was in keeping with the wider ambulance service with 64 per cent indicating they were men. The age distribution showed that the majority (68 per cent) were under the age of 41. A large number of respondents were from metropolitan centres with only 7.4 per cent of respondents indicating that they were based in rural or regional areas. Most respondents didn't care where their experience was from or what sort of experience it was as long as they had valid roadside experience. What mattered was that the values of the clinical leaders were matched by their actions and abilities. Many did not see themselves as clinical leaders and most thought they could not influence organisational issues. Most respondents thought they should have an influence on clinical care and valued team working. Clinical leaders (in keeping with the previous study) were seen to be visible role models, leaders in clinical practice, skilled, experienced, clinically focused, approachable, knowledgeable, driven by their desire to provide high-quality care, and have a high moral character and change practice. They were seen to be team members who made decisions often under pressure.

STUDY 3   LEADERSHIP AT HOME: PERCEPTIONS OF CLINICAL LEADERSHIP AT SWAN CARE GROUP BENTLEY PARK

Aim: To investigate perceptions of leadership and approaches to leadership development of senior nurses and care home managers in an aged care residential facility in Western Australia.

Location: Swan Care residential facility in Bentley Park, Perth, Western Australia.

Dates: March – September 2012.

Methodology: Qualitative – phenomenology methods – questionnaire and interviews.

Target group: Senior clinical nurses and residential care home managers in one residential care home in Western Australia.

Analysis: Interviews = NVivo 0.6 and manual data configuration questionnaire = SPSS.

Sample: 20 staff were sent questionnaires: 10 were returned (rate of = 50 per cent). Eight senior nurses or care home staff were interviewed (some had also completed the questionnaire).

Gender mix: Questionnaires: Female = 100 per cent / Male = 0 per cent; Interviews: Female = 100 per cent / Male = 0 per cent.

Ethics: Ethical approval was sought and secured with the University of Western Australia Human Research Ethics Office (RA/4/1/5084) and the study had the consent of the management of Swan Care Bentley Park.

Results: The attributes and characteristics of clinical leaders identified by the senior nurses and care home managers who participated in the study were consistent with the results of the two previous studies, with the vast majority of respondents suggesting that clinical leaders were identified because they were approachable, had sound clinical skills and knowledge, were honest, had integrity, supported others and were visible in the clinical area. It was also noted that participants saw a distinction between leadership and management and that their more clinically focused roles led them toward a leadership-centred approach. However, few had any leadership instruction beyond clinical 'experience' and almost all saw barriers that hindered their development or application of leadership in the care home environment. In order to play a more effective part in service improvement and care provision with a positive impact on resident care and staff support, it was considered essential that senior nursing and care home managers be better supported in recognising the significance of developing clinical leadership attributes and applying them in the care home environment.

As with the two previous studies, few participants saw themselves as clinical leaders, although they recognised that clinical leaders were evident at all levels in the care home. The 'manager' was less likely to be seen as a clinical leader than the more senior clinically focused nursing staff. As with the previous studies, the attribute least

(Continued)

(Continued)

likely to be associated with clinical leadership was 'controlling' (80 per cent). Again, leaders seemed to be recognised because they had their values on show rather than because of any affinity with their vision.

STUDY 4   VOLUNTEER AMBULANCE OFFICERS' PERCEPTIONS OF CLINICAL LEADERSHIP IN ST JOHN AMBULANCE SERVICES WESTERN AUSTRALIA INC.

Aim: To investigate the perceptions of leadership and approaches to the application of clinical leadership with Volunteer Ambulance Officers (VAO) in the St John Ambulance Services in Western Australia.

Location: Western Australia (metropolitan, rural and remote areas of practice).

Dates: September 2012 – April 2013.

Methodology: Qualitative – phenomenology methods – online and paper-based questionnaires were used.

Target group: Volunteer Ambulance Officers (VAOs) in Western Australia.

Analysis: Questionnaire (paper-based and online) with SPSS.

Sample: Approximately 500 volunteer ambulance officers were sent questionnaires (although there were estimated to be 2,787 VAOs in the WA service at the time of the study); 61 were returned, a return rate of only 12.2 per cent.

Gender mix: Questionnaire: Female = 49 per cent / Male = 51 per cent.

Ethics: Ethical approval was sought and secured with the University of Western Australia Human Research Ethics Office (RA/4/1/5451) and had the consent of the management of the St John Ambulance Service WA Inc was secured.

Results: Only 32.7 per cent indicated that they had some sort of formal leadership training (although it was not clear what this constituted). A further 60.7 per cent indicated that they had not had any formal leadership training and 6.6 per cent were not sure. In terms of formal management training a similar 31.2 per cent indicated that they had had some sort of management training while 65.5 per cent indicated that they had not, with 3.3 per cent unsure. The gender make-up of the respondents was interesting in that there was almost a 50:50 split with men making up 50.8 per cent of the sample and women making up the remainder. A large number of respondents were from regional centres with only 8.2 per cent of respondents indicating that they were based in the metropolitan areas.

In relation to the characteristics of a clinical leader, most suggested that clinical leaders needed to be clinically competent (90 per cent), a role model for others (89 per cent) and an effective communicator (87 per cent) as well as to inspire confidence (85 per cent), to be approachable (84 per cent), to have integrity (79 per cent), to be flexible (77 per cent) and to set direction (75 per cent). Almost 84 per cent indicated (in keeping with all the studies) that 'controlling' was the attribute least associated with clinical leadership. Most didn't care where their experience was from or what sort of experience it was as long as they had valid roadside experience. What mattered was that the values of the clinical leaders were matched by their actions and abilities. Many respondents did not see themselves as clinical leaders and few thought they could influence organisational issues. Most thought they should have an influence on clinical care and valued team working. In keeping with their paramedic colleagues, clinical leaders were seen to be visible role models, leaders in clinical practice, skilled, experienced, clinically focused, approachable, knowledgeable, driven by their desire to provide high-quality care, have high moral character and change practice. They were seen to be team members who made decisions often under pressure.

STUDY 5   WESTERN AUSTRALIAN ALLIED HEALTH PROFESSIONALS' PERCEPTIONS OF CLINICAL LEADERSHIP

Aim: To identify how the concept and application of clinical leadership is perceived by allied health professionals (AHPs) and the implications for service improvement, the adoption of quality initiatives and innovations for change.

Location: Western Australia (metropolitan, rural and remote areas of practice).

Dates: November/December 2014.

Methodology: Mixed methods with quantitative data dominating the mix methods – online SurveyMonkey questionnaire.

Target group: Allied Health Professionals employed within the Western Australian Department of Health. Main professional disciplines included dietetics, occupational therapy, physiotherapy, podiatry, social work and speech pathology.

Analysis: Questionnaire = SPSS (version 21) with qualitative data analysed by spreadsheet and Word documents.

Sample size: 311 online questionnaires were returned with 307 offering relevant data.

Gender mix: Female = 86.5 per cent / Male = 13.5 per cent.

Ethics: Ethical approval was sought and secured through the Government of Western Australian Department of Health, South Metropolitan Health Service, Human Research Ethics Committee (No.: HREC 14/45 Code: EC00265).

Results: Participants in this study represented only 6.1 per cent of the total AHP workforce of the Western Australian Department of Health. The data indicated that

(Continued)

(Continued)

the respondents had been AHPs for an average of 14.6 years. The vast majority of respondents came from the six targeted allied health professional groups of: dietetics (11.2 per cent), occupational therapy (17.8 per cent), physiotherapy (19.7 per cent), podiatry (3.0 per cent), social work (18.4 per cent) and speech pathology (15.5 per cent). The majority of respondents were at Health Service Union Award (HSU) Level P1 (base grade clinician) or P2 (senior clinician) (68.1 per cent) with only about 15 per cent of respondents being at Level P4 or beyond. The majority of respondents (86.5 per cent) were female and the median respondent age was 38.9 years, with the majority of AHP respondents being between 21 and 40 (54.3 per cent). In addition, the majority of respondents worked in acute hospital environments (59.9 per cent) and in a metropolitan location (73.7 per cent).

In terms of the respondents' perceptions of clinical leadership, the majority of respondents (79.2 per cent) saw themselves, and thought they were seen by others (76.2 per cent), as clinical leaders. The main attributes identified as being attributed to clinical leaders were: is an effective communicator, sets direction, is clinically competent, has integrity and is honest, is approachable, acts as a role model for others, copes well with change, is supportive, is a mentor and is a motivator. The main attributes identified as being least associated with a clinical leader was 'is controlling' (83.7 per cent). In support of this, when asked if a clinical leader needed to be in a management position to be effective only 22.2 per cent agreed they did. However, when asked if having a clinical focus was important for an effective clinical leader, 85.3 per cent suggested it was. Other attributes seen as central for effective clinical leadership were having the skills and resources to perform tasks effectively, having teamworking skills, being visible in the clinical environment, expressing appreciation to colleagues, being an initiator, having a high moral character, communicating well or being an 'excellent communicator' and being flexible.

Clinical leaders were also perceived as having an impact on how clinical care is delivered, supporting staff, being innovative, leading change and service improvement, participating in professional development and (although to a lesser extent) influencing organisational policy. A large number of respondents (81.4 per cent) indicated that there were barriers hindering their effectiveness as clinical leaders. The barriers included: a lack of time and a high clinical demand on their time, having to deal with bureaucracy, a lack of opportunities to be a clinical leader, limited funding and resources, a lack of mentorship, working part-time and problems with the whole health system.

STUDY 6   CLINICAL LEADERSHIP PERCEPTIONS OF RURAL AND REMOTE AREA NURSES IN NORTH-WESTERN NSW

Aim: To identify how the concepts and application of clinical leadership are perceived by rural and remote area nurses in North-Western New South Wales, Australia.

Location: North- Western New South Wales, Australia (rural and remote areas of practice).

Dates: September/November 2017.

Methodology: Phenomenological/qualitative methods – interviews.

Target group: Rural and remote area nurses (RNs and ENs) in remote clinics and small rural or remote hospitals across North-Western NSW, Australia.

Analysis: Questionnaire = SPSS (version 21) with qualitative data analysed by spreadsheet and Word documents.

Sample Size: 56 interviews.

Gender mix: Female = 90 per cent / Male = 10 per cent.

Ethics: Ethical approval was sought and secured through the Hunter New England Human Research Ethics Committee of Hunter New England Local Health District, (Reference 17/06/21/5.02).

Results: Thematic analysis led to 5 themes: Leadership in rural and remote areas; The impact of clinical leadership in rural and remote areas; Barriers in rural and remote practice; Training and development challenges; and Rural and remote practice challenges. Findings suggested that clinical leadership is understood and character- ised in much the same way as it is in studies in other Australian and international clinical environments. As well, clinical leaders were seen to have a significant impact on the quality of care and initiation of change. However, they also faced barriers if the health facility was poorly staffed, lacked support and if the community were strongly co-dependent. This gave disproportionate power to staff who had close relationships in the community and longevity in the clinical facility. This hinted at real challenges when addressing a culture of safety and changes in practices if these were at odds with the way things had always been done in the health facility. The clinical leaders' attributes were in keeping with all of the previous studies.

The results from the studies outlined above have led to the development of the leadership theory **Congruent Leadership** outlined in this book. This theory suggests that clinical leaders demonstrate a match (congruence) between the leader's values and beliefs and their actions.

The research results indicated that clinically focused nurses and a range of health professionals that have moved decisively and clearly in the direction of their values and beliefs can be seen to be expressing Congruent Leadership. They may have simply stood by their values, working not because they wanted to change the world but because they knew that what they were doing was the right thing and their actions were making a difference.

When acting out or role modelling their values and beliefs (even subconsciously) something was happening in their relationships with their clients, patients or col- leagues that gave a clear signal about what they believed, or what their values were.

This links Congruent Leadership with the expression of emotional intelligence and values-based relationship building.

The research studies indicate that others, responding to the expression of the leaders' values and beliefs in action, saw these leaders as such because they were approachable, clinically knowledgeable and competent. They were visible in practice, role models for the practice they espouse and communicated well. They were able to make effective decisions, were empowered and could motivate others, and because their actions were evident or matched their values and beliefs they were seen as passionate and committed leaders. It was rarely because they were visionaries, in powerful positions or wielded great authority.

The studies were undertaken with a range of different health professionals, used a range of methodologies, were undertaken in different countries or across the scope of one large country, addressed different genders and took place over a wide span of years. The study results have been presented in a number of countries (e.g. Thailand, Singapore, Tanzania, Canada, the UK, the USA, Australia and Ireland), all with resounding endorsements of the principles of Congruent Leadership theory. In addition, three replica studies are underway in the UK, Australia and South Africa.

Each of the six completed studies outlined above were focused on capturing data about clinically focused leaders; however, the results point to a new way of understanding leadership that suggests that leaders are followed, not for being visionary, for being creative or for being transformational, but because there is a match between their values and beliefs and how these are translated into their actions.

These clinically focused leaders capture what it means to be a congruent leader – standing by their values in the execution and drive of their actions, putting their hands where their hearts are, walking their walk and acting out and following through with what they believe to be right. These leaders are not selling a vision or communicating a path for others to follow, they are living their values and walking the path themselves, role modelling with commitment, conviction and determination what they believe is the right thing to do. They are congruent leaders.

Congruent leaders demonstrate where their values lie and are followed because others identify with these same values and stand with them. Congruent leaders are followed when others have respect for or connect with the leader's values as demonstrated in their actions. In an example from another professional group, firefighters will follow fellow firefighters who are knowledgeable about the duties and responsibilities of their work, who care for their own and others' safety, who act as team members and don't put others' lives at risk. They are followed if they are role models for teamwork, safety, courage, strength or stamina and show commitment to the other members of their team. Firefighters who communicate well, are seen to behave in keeping with these values and are seen as a cohesive part of the team may be followed even without the title of team leader or being in a senior or managerial position. Other firefighters identify with these values and behaviours and with the firefighter's capacity to empathise with colleagues. Leaders like this are not followed because they were born to lead, have a titled position, have a vision or have authority over others. They are followed because they put their values and beliefs into action and others recognise an alignment of their own values with those of the leader.

A SOLID FOUNDATION

Congruent Leadership establishes a foundation from which all effective leadership can start, because it grounds the leader's principles within the core values of their personal, professional or work role principles and values. This will ensure that the dominant cultural narrative of these personal, professional or work role principles and values are evident in this person's actions. In this way, the person's core values are placed front and centre and act as a foundation on which to build their engagement with the organisation, their colleagues and customers or service users.

The recognition and application of Congruent Leadership may offer organisations an opportunity to develop leaders who can exercise greater influence over the productivity and success of the organisation. This is because congruent leaders foster a focus on the organisation's values, as long as these are made explicit and as long as employees, workers, staff, etc. are willing to support and promote these values. If the organisation's espoused values are adrift from the reality of the organisation's actions the foundation is threatened. Enron (a once massive American energy company) had the following core values: Communication, Respect, Excellence and Integrity. These were stated in their annual reports and posted on the organisation's walls. However, these were not role modelled or seen in action and as such they failed to form a firm foundation for the company to be built upon or grow. Enron is now a byword for organisational corruption and slippage of values.

If the 'lived values' of an organisation are in conflict with the organisation's 'espoused values', members of the organisation will feel in conflict. This type of 'clash of values' has been found to disrupt the development, success and performance of companies in the business world (O'Reilly and Pfeffer, 2000) and in my own experience in the health service I have seen this 'clash' many times. Generally, clinically focused health professionals at the 'coal face' of patient care are driven by their professional values to provide quality, compassionate care and to deal with people's needs in a timely and effective way. However, if they are working in a resource-poor or financially constrained organisation, or if the organisation is focused on delivering different values, their professional values may be compromised.

This can occur to the point where the organisation takes a dim view of the very professional or employee values that the professionals or employees were recruited to deliver in the first place. If professionals or employees work in organisations where they are unable or inhibited from expressing their core values and beliefs, negative consequences follow. These negative implications can occur on a raft of levels. The quality of services may fall, staff may become disenchanted or disengaged further affecting services. Staff may leave or stay, perform poorly or even sabotage the organisation. Organisations, businesses, institutions, etc. may react by resorting to systems and processes because they are easier to initiate than dealing with 'culture' which rests on values. The aim is to try to exert greater control and authority; however, the net effect is often to drive the core professional or employee values further from the focus of the organisational culture.

Congruent leaders help ground the values and beliefs of an organisation. As such, their leadership impact is likely to be considerable, either in favour of the organisation's espoused values or in support of the employee's professional values (hopefully both if they are aligned correctly). If there is a match, then the impact of the congruent leader can be very powerful (this theme is taken up further in Chapter 7).

SCENARIO 2.1   CONGRUENT LEADERSHIP IN ACTION

Two physiotherapists had been working on a medical rehabilitation ward in a busy city hospital. Each had for some years been following a practice by which all patients with cardiac problems had to demonstrate that they could climb a set of stairs prior to discharge. This had become a pre-discharge prerequisite and no person with cardiac problems could be discharged until this task had been demonstrated and recorded. The issue the physiotherapists identified was that often this meant a patient's discharge was delayed (commonly over weekends) until a physiotherapist could supervise this activity.

They undertook to identify where the practice had originated and what clinical evidence sat behind the practice. They met with all the cardiac medical officers in the hospital and consulted a wide range of literature. The literature proved of limited value and the medical staff even less so, as they suggested the practice had not originated with them.

Faced with a practice that seemed to have no basis in clinical evidence or medical practice the two physiotherapists suggested that it served no sound clinical purpose and that it should be stopped. While clearly offering a number of benefits to the hospital in terms of reducing length of stay and speeding discharge processes, the hospital and ward managers were at first not keen to change the practice. The managers were not sure that a change, initiated as it was by two physiotherapists, was worthy of consideration. The managers were concerned that not all medical practitioners were in favour of the change and they thought there must be a good reason for it as 'it had been going on for so long'.

The physiotherapists persisted and recruited key medical staff to argue their position. They knew that a change to a less specific cardiac assessment would result in better outcomes for the patients, the assessment process and the discharge issues, and because of these factors they were resolute and determined.

The physiotherapists had been motivated to identify this change in practice because they valued better, more effective and evidence-based outcomes for the people with cardiac problems. The physiotherapists used excellent communication skills and were seen as collaborative and collegial by their medical partners and the outcome was soon a better, more flexible and appropriate assessment strategy that allowed many more patients access to a speedier and safe discharge. These physiotherapists were congruent leaders, acting on and putting into practice their values about taking steps to support better client care.

CONGRUENT LEADERSHIP AND QUALITY

During an induction or orientation to any organisation, it is common to hear that 'quality is everyone's business'. Indeed it is, although in practice quality is sometimes seen as nobody's business. The challenge for many organisations is to effectively engage all employees and staff in quality processes and it is in this area that congruent leaders may be able to make a significant contribution.

As the emphasis on quality increases, it is becoming imperative that front-line, coalface, service desk, bedside and front-of-house staff or employees are engaged in driving or supporting the quality agenda across the organisation. This can be supported further if all levels of staff or employees are encouraged to recognise themselves as stakeholders in the industry, institution or organisation in which they work. These staff or employees can do so much more if they are recognised (by themselves and others) as leaders in the area of quality and encouraged to see that leadership does indeed exist at many levels. If all staff can display Congruent Leadership and if their passion for participation in quality processes and service improvement can be enhanced. The result will be a greater pool from which role models for quality improvement and quality service can be drawn.

If all levels of employees or staff focus on the values that are central to their work role they will also be drawn towards focusing on improving service provision and quality processes. It is clear that safety and quality issues are of paramount importance in all organisations. Therefore, activating or supporting a host of 'grassroots' level staff or employees to role model or 'champion' appropriate safety and quality activities and processes will go further than issuing memos and posting periodic reminders about safety. It is proposed here that the key to impacting most effectively on safety and quality processes is to focus on the development of leadership skills at all levels, but specifically on leaders who function at the 'coalface' of the organisation and those in close proximity to service users, customers and key points of production.

Congruent leaders are those who operate in daily contact with clients and patients, customers, service users and the public, and they are more likely to recognise and be able to respond to deficits in services or lapses in quality. If organisations and institutions are to deliver safe, high-quality services or products then governance systems and processes need to be robust and operate throughout the organisation. For this to be the case, communication systems and leadership systems need to be robust and acknowledge the critical place that 'grassroots' congruent leaders play in implementing quality processes or reporting faults in quality processes.

The UK NHS National Patient Safety Agency (2004) suggests seven steps for ensuring patient safety, with 'lead and support' for staff as the second step. However, this can be most effectively implemented if the leadership is in keeping with core organisational values and provided by staff who are placed in view of those required to engage in quality work. In this way quality becomes part of what staff or employees see being role modelled by congruent leaders who are visible and engaged at the coalface, shopfloor, bedside, etc. This implies that it is 'grassroots' leaders with Congruent Leadership skills and attributes that are best placed to ensure safety and quality processes. Similarly, in Australia the Victorian Quality Council (2005) suggested that bedside (clinically focused) leaders play a significant role in quality processes by participating in the setting of strategic safety objectives and taking responsibility for implementing the safety agenda. This is no different to any industry or organisation. They also suggest that bedside leaders should support the allocation of resources to promote best practice (Victorian Quality Council, 2005). They should act as 'champions' for service improvement (Victorian Quality Council, 2005). They should raise the status of safety and quality activities, contribute to clinically focused improvement initiatives and educate their fellow clinicians with training support for further engagement with safety and quality activities (Victorian Quality Council, 2005). Mahoney (2001) and Rich (2008) support these suggestions and add that bedside health professional leaders (of any discipline) should act as role models for quality, provide expert evidence-based care, collaborate with others to facilitate best practice, take responsibility for quality initiatives and advocate for changes that will benefit service users (clients and patients).

If these aspirations are central to how congruent leaders practice or act, then Congruent Leadership will be evident in supporting or promoting quality improvement. Indeed, it is argued that it is because front-line, coalface, service desk, bedside and front-of-house staff may be driven by their values and beliefs that these leaders, displaying Congruent Leadership, are ideally placed to impact positively on safety and quality processes.

ACTIVITY 2.1   REFLECTIVE EXERCISE

- What are your values?
- At work …
- At home …

Are they different? Does this matter? Are your values the same as those of your partners or colleagues? Find out by asking them what their values are.

CONGRUENT LEADERSHIP AND POWER

Congruent Leadership is not power neutral. The power of Congruent Leadership comes from unifying groups and individuals around common values and beliefs. This is not a strategy as such, but the results from my research studies appear to demonstrate that people seek out or follow leaders who are more inclined to display or hold values and beliefs that they themselves hold. A front-line, coalface, bedside, chalk-side, service desk and front-of-house employee operating within a clear set of values or core principles is more likely to be recognised as a person to follow than a person who functions outside of the organisation's values or guiding principles, or who is not directly engaged in the work functions associated with the employee.

Therefore an office worker whose values and beliefs are consistent with the dominant values and beliefs of their colleagues or the organisation will find they are seen as a leader (if they apply their values and beliefs to their actions) or will be able to exercise more effective leadership by virtue of this alignment. They may not know they are seen as a leader and they may not be seeking to lead. However, the alignment of their values and beliefs with their actions will position them to be able to bring their colleagues to a point where their values and beliefs coincide. Conflict can result if the principles and values of one individual or group are at odds with others and power and influence in terms of leading falls often to the dominant group or leader.

A congruent leader's power and influence is derived from being able to articulate and display their values, beliefs and principles, with actions being more effective in getting a message across than words. Followers recognise or align themselves with these same values or beliefs and by supporting and promoting them, increase the leader's credibility and worth. By promoting the significance of 'this' leader's values and beliefs over any others, the leader would be able to influence or change practice or generate innovation. Change, although often not the intention, results when values and beliefs are displayed, promoted and then adopted by the followers.

Some of the world's most powerful leaders have been congruent leaders. They were followed because they were able to articulate and display their values and beliefs. Their values and beliefs resonated with many people and their ability to influence (in many cases millions of people) is truly awesome. Buddha, Confucius, Jesus and Muhammad were in effect congruent leaders. Powerful leadership is evident when leaders respond to challenges and critical problems with actions and activities in accord with, or congruent with, their values and beliefs. However, Congruent Leadership is seldom exercised by people in positions of control or authority. Power and control commonly negate the impact of values and the element of choice, which is vital for followers of congruent leaders, is lost.

CONGRUENT LEADERSHIP AND INNOVATION/CHANGE

Gandhi said, 'We must be the change we wish to see in the world.' In many ways this sits as the core of what Congruent Leadership means. In the studies used to expose Congruent Leadership, no assumptions were made about who the clinical leaders were or what their characteristics might be; instead, these matters were rigorously explored. Recognising the significance of values and beliefs and their impact on actions is vital, but in terms of influencing innovation and change it is also essential that leaders understand the tools that can be used to facilitate change.

Sometimes change or innovation is slow or resisted because people have not considered or learnt to listen to their 'true' or inner voice. It may also be that they have not learned the skills associated with effectively managing or driving change and innovation or the liberation of empowerment. The ideas and suggestions for change are there – just listen into any tearoom or lunch table or water cooler conversation. It may also be that many people are not clear about what leadership means, but they can be leaders or are recognised as leaders in the workplace, office, school, health facility or factory.

While managers might have the authority to support change, they may not have the workplace focus or practical insights to see what change is needed at the coalface or where the work is done. Thus it is employees and staff at the 'grassroots' of an organisation who are in an ideal position to see the change that is needed, and the value and impact change and innovations can have on production or services. Conceptualised in this way the ideal leaders are not managers, but employees at any level of an organisation, although, sadly, in many organisations they may feel they lack the authority to take their ideas and suggestions further.

Change and innovation can be affected by the congruent leader. First, though, the congruent leader needs to understand the significance of their own values and beliefs. Second, they need to recognise that they have followers, because these followers have recognised a match between the leader's values and beliefs and their actions. In the initial study, described in Study 1, it was very common for leaders identified as such by their colleagues to say 'What me? Don't you want to talk to my manager?' People, it seems, often look to leaders for leadership, even if the leader isn't aware of it. The third point is that change can occur even without power or formal authority, if leaders can learn to use reflection, change management techniques or strategies, to employ creativity, evidence-based approaches and networks, and to delegate effectively. This can be achieved without formal authority or hierarchical power. Finally, for congruent leaders bringing about change and innovation they will need to motivate and inspire others and minimise the change killer, namely conflict.

Congruent leaders exercise their values-based influence on change and support innovation if they are able to recognise that leadership is not tied to positions of power, titles, badges, big offices and authority, or if they can see that leaders do not need to have the 'big picture' or 'vision' or be in powerful authoritarian positions or hold budgetary control. In fact, it can be congruent leaders in front-line, coalface, roadside, bedside and factory-floor positions (Stanton et al., 2010) that can bring about meaningful and significant change, simply by doing what they feel is the 'right' thing. Then, when they employ (or can learn to employ) collaborative strategies to limit conflict, develop the motivation and influence of others and change management techniques or strategies, they can be the force that will help an organisation, institution, industry or business deliver high-quality, high-production or great service that will shape a better tomorrow for the organisation, its products and services.

EXAMPLES OF CONGRUENT LEADERS

Not all congruent leaders are recognised as leaders in the way many management or even leadership texts might describe them. Rosa Parks was an African American woman on a bus in Montgomery, Alabama in 1955. She was on her way home from work. While she was already a civil rights activist working for the National Association for the Advancement of Colored People (NAACP), she had not deliberately set out to change the world with her actions on the bus that day. She was tired and simply wanted to get home. She was sitting on a seat on a bus when a white man wanted her seat. Parks refused to give up her seat and was arrested under racially motivated laws. Later when asked to explain why she didn't give up her seat she said simply, 'Our mistreatment was just not right, and I was tired of it.' Here was a congruent leader who stood up (sat) for her values and beliefs, and by simply acting on her values and beliefs became the figurehead for the American Civil Rights movement. This was not the planned action of a radical trying to rebel against the law. There was nothing predetermined in her actions. She did what she felt was the right thing to do, to assert the values she displayed in other areas of her life, both personal and professional, in the face of unjust and immoral laws. In this act she had her values on show: she was courageous, empowered and visible as she made her stand.

Two other people who stood by their values and became leaders were Betty Williams and Mairead Corrigan, mothers and housewives from Belfast, Ireland. They have each been recognised for their desire to end violence in Northern Ireland. However, their path of leadership was a tragic one when in August 1976 a car driven by an IRA gunman who had been shot fleeing British soldiers crashed into a family group on a quiet residential street in Belfast. The 'troubles' in Northern Ireland had been particularly bloody and deadly in 1976, but the death of two children outright (a third died later from injuries sustained) and the wounding of their mother motivated Betty and Mairead to act.

Betty, who had witnessed the accident as she drove home, and Mairead, who was related to the children killed in the crash, were so appalled by the incident and ongoing violence that within a short time they had collected a mass of signatures to petition the British government for an end to the strife. This led to them establishing the Community of Peace that aimed to unite and build positive relationships between Protestants and Catholics in Northern Ireland.

Both women were instrumental (with the support of Ciaran McKeown from the Northern Ireland Press) in bringing the conflicted factions together. They set up summer camps for mixed groups of children in a number of European countries and put pressure on their communities and government to unite around values of peace and non-violence. Their values were summed up in Betty's acceptance speech when they received the Nobel Peace Prize in 1979. In it she said:

> We have a simple message for the world from this movement for peace. We want to live and love and build a just and peaceful society. We want for our children, as we want for ourselves, our lives at home, at work and at play, to be lives of joy and peace. We recognise that to build such a life demands of all of us dedication, hard work and courage … We dedicate ourselves to working with our neighbours, near and far, day in and day out, to building that peaceful society in which the tragedies we have known are a bad memory and a continuing warning.

Their immediate response to the tragic car crash was to unite the press and community in support of their values. Since then Betty and Mairead have travelled the world, supporting peaceful solutions to other conflicts and arranging protests against injustice and political repression. They continue to speak out about how their values shaped their actions and how their actions forged a new reality in Northern Ireland. The values of these two extraordinary 'ordinary' people show what anyone can accomplish if they harness the power of their values (peace, joy, love and non-violence) by acting on them with determination and courage.

CHAPTER SUMMARY

This chapter has outlined a new leadership theory called Congruent Leadership. The theory grew from the results of a number of substantial research projects undertaken between 2001 and 2018 that set out to specifically explore leadership in the health service. Congruent Leadership is proposed as a framework to support an understanding of leadership from a 'grassroots' perspective. Congruent Leadership offers a solid foundation for novice leaders to gain leadership potential and understand a new perspective on leadership.

Congruent Leadership is defined as a match (congruence) between the values and beliefs of the leader and their actions. These types of leader are evident at any level within an organisation, although they are commonly not seen where the leader exercises authority or control. Congruent leaders are found in great numbers across the spectrum of any organisation, institution or business. Congruent leaders have stepped boldly in the direction of their values and beliefs or confidently stood by them, sometimes in spite of opposition or conflict. Congruent leaders are not selling a vision or communicating a path for others to follow. They are living their values and walking their paths with conviction, commitment and determination.

Congruent leadership is not power neutral. The power of Congruent Leadership comes from unifying groups and individuals around common values and beliefs. If leaders (at any level) focus on the values that are central to their profession, industry, business or organisation, they will draw others onto focusing on improving the core aspects of their profession, industry, business or organisation with a direct impact on improving quality and bringing about change or innovation. In this way, congruent leaders are focused on innovation and change by acting out their values and beliefs.

3

ATTRIBUTES OF CONGRUENT LEADERS

'Sometimes one pays most for the things one gets for nothing.'

Albert Einstein, theoretical physicist

INTRODUCTION

This chapter outlines the attributes and characteristics that may be attributed to congruent leaders and as identified from the research studies outlined in the preceding chapter. In doing so this chapter further clarifies the parameters for understanding how to recognise a congruent leader within your practice because, as discussed, they are not always marked out by a smart office or a fancy title, but may be working side by side with you. The chapter concludes by exploring examples of who congruent leaders might be and outlines the implications for understanding and recognising leaders, who lead by matching the values and beliefs with their actions.

CONGRUENT LEADERSHIP ATTRIBUTES

Attempts to describe the attributes of leaders are not new. Many, many others have explored leadership by trying to define or describe the attributes, characteristics and abilities of leaders. Indeed, this forms the basis of the 'Trait Theory' of leadership. I began my own journey to discover more about leadership by exploring the attributes of clinical leaders, commonly leaders who lead without formal power or authority and in many respects it was this exploration that pointed towards and supported my insights into Congruent Leadership.

CONGRUENT LEADER ATTRIBUTES OUTLINED

There are ten key attributes evident in congruent leaders. These are:

1. Values on show (passionate/doer/persistent/determined/dynamic/energetic/positive)
2. Approachable (open)
3. Charismatic/inspirational/motivational
4. Visible/role model
5. Courageous (confident/consistent/reliable)
6. Good communicator (calm/good listener)
7. Empathetic
8. Competent/knowledgeable/good decision-maker
9. Empowered
10. Honesty (integrity/trustworthy)

The development of insights into these attributes has come about from studying clinical leaders, but they can be translated into attributes for leaders in any field, industry, organisation or business and any walk of life. Many of the attributes are interrelated and interdependent so that it would be unusual if a congruent leader, who was considered approachable, was not also visible, empathetic and a good communicator. However, each of these attributes has been singled out and will be explored separately as a way of establishing a complete map of congruent leader attributes.

─────────────── **ACTIVITY 3.1   REFLECTIVE EXERCISE** ───────────────

Look at the list above.

Do you recognise any of these in terms of your own clinical practice or professional role? How are they expressed in what you do at work or in the clinical/practice domain?

───

We will now explore each of these attributes in further detail.

1. **Values on show (passionate/doer/persistent/determined/dynamic/energetic/positive)**

   Congruent leaders are followed because others recognise them for living out their values in the things they do. As such doing nothing (although this too reflects a value set) is seldom something that would point towards being recognised as a congruent leader. People who apply themselves to the things they do with passion and positivity, who are dynamic and determined or persistently driven to strive toward the embodiment of their values in the things they do, are congruent leaders. Above all, congruent leaders are doers, actors on the stage of their life, walking down the path laid out by the values they hold. They step forward or stand by their values boldly, passionately, persistently and with determination. They are energetic and dynamic in doing what is central to their beliefs and support the things they believe are the right things to do. As such, their values are on show.

Sometimes (in fact often) this occurs unconsciously. Not all congruent leaders are able to verbalise or describe what their values are. However, they know and do what they feel is the right thing to do.

2. Approachable (open)

Congruent leaders are commonly approachable. Being open and transparent with people, allowing others to see what they believe, means trusting people and being trusted. Trusting others and risking acceptance or rejection, but being open and trusting anyway, means allowing others to have access to them. If leaders are not open or approachable, people will be unable to get close enough to see what the leader is doing and they will be unable to clearly recognise the values the leader has. This will in turn lead to a lack of trust and diminish the leader's ability to effectively relate to others. Being friendly, approachable and understanding means that potential followers feel valued or important, and that leaders are there for them. Approachability also opens the door for a two-way conversation and greater mutual understanding, vital if values are to be clearly translated and understood.

3. Charismatic/inspirational/motivational

This is a delicate attribute as so many negative assumptions are attributed to charismatic approaches to leadership. Rafferty (1993, p. 8) sees charisma as a 'potentially exploitative' aspect of leadership while others align charismatic leaders with control and spiritual or personal influence, used to manipulate their followers. The Jonestown incident with Jim Jones leading hundreds of people to take part in a mass suicide in 1978, or the events of the Waco siege in 1993 where the Branch Davidians led by David Koresh held out against the FBI for 51 days and resulted in the deaths of 76 people, are examples of the power of charisma at its worst. 'Charisma' is itself hard to define making it something that many leadership authors shy away from. In relation to Congruent Leadership it is aligned with being approachable and positive, even passionate about living out their values. Charisma here is aligned with being inspirational. Inspiration is described as an arousal of the mind to a special or unusual activity or creativity, or the arousal of a particular emotion or action. These are the effects of effective Congruent Leadership, with followers being stimulated or inspired to do or act in ways that change what they have been doing, because they see the values of the leader embodied in the actions of the leader. As in the examples above, charisma can have a powerful impact on the application of values into action even if they have negative consequences. Goleman et al. (2013) view leaders who can inspire as being able to articulate a shared set of values that resonate with and motivate others.

This may require charisma, that 'special power' that some people have, or it may take an ability to simply, persistently and determinedly continue to act out and live by the values that the leader holds to be appropriate and it is the 'doing' involved in living out their values that motivates or inspires others.

4. Visible/role model

Being visible is vital if congruent leaders are to be effective. Followers look to congruent leaders who put their values into practice. They 'walk the walk' of their values and if these cannot be seen then followers will be disconnected from the central focus of the leader's influence.

In being visible congruent leaders are also available and present. To be visible is to be present, to be 'around' and to be 'there' for others. It is not helpful if leaders are not available to directly guide followers and it is not possible to put the leader's values into action if they are simply not there to do so. This can be time-consuming and even exhausting. It asks that the leader give something of themselves and there is a tangible cost to leading in this way. If congruent leaders are to be visible it means they are required to be present in the environment in which they lead, not just that they are seen to be there but that they are actively engaged and involved.

Being engaged and visible also implies that the congruent leader is competent, knowledgeable, able to communicate effectively, make effective decisions and is empowered and motivational. This means they are open and approachable and acting as a role model. Not being visible or being unable to be involved in the workplace or group activity may be seen by some to place the leader in a difficult position, or one that weakens their leadership potential or credibility.

However, being visible means that congruent leaders are able to role model not just their values, but also the attributes of effective leadership. Their values are visible, they have their standards of behaviour and ways to actively be involved and on show. Recognising this, others lend their support to the congruent leader's ability to both lead and to role model the attributes of this type of leader. In keeping with the ideal of Gandhi's quote, congruent leaders are being the 'change they wish to see in the world'.

5. Courageous (confident/consistent/reliable)

Remaining true to your values is not always easy. History is replete with examples of people who have been persecuted and ridiculed for holding fast to what they thought were the right things to do. Many people have stood firm in the face of abuse, rejection, isolation, punishment and even death. This sort of leadership takes great courage. Benazir Bhutto, Dr Martin Luther King and Rosa Parks are just a few examples of people who risked much to hold fast to the values they held dear and the beliefs that sustained them.

This type of fortitude requires a consistent and persistent application of the leader's values. The leader needs to be seen to apply their values with consistency and not vacillate in the face of opposition or criticism. When Julia Gillard, Prime Minister of Australia (2010–13), took forward a policy that attempted to address climate change that was not popular, she faced determined and sometimes vicious personal abuse from colleagues and the political opposition, but she courageously held true to the values and principles she believed were ultimately in the best interests of the future of Australia's climate.

This type of leadership means that courage is expressed as a consistent approach to the things the leader does (and says) and that people can count on the leader to be reliable, even in the face of opposition and criticism. Standing by our values – doing 'the right thing' – is rarely easy, and it demands more of the leader than pointing in the direction of a vision and asking others to 'trust me', to 'go forth and deliver'. It is the test of our own beliefs and convictions, and in some cases this type of leadership comes with great risks. Mahatma Gandhi faced down the government in South Africa during the non-violent, civil disobedience campaign between 1906 and 1913, an example of a congruent leader in action. Gandhi took part, he was visible, he was at the head of the protests and he suffered through his actions alongside the followers of the movement. Congruent leaders need to be very courteous.

6. Good communicator (calm/good listener)

Congruent leaders do not need to be great orators. It cannot hurt of course, but the key to effective congruent leadership from a communication perspective rests more in being able to listen and remain calm rather than talk. The central aspect of communicating is through the congruent leader's actions. People will see and recognise the leader's values through what they do. Therefore, it is not essential for a congruent leader to be able to describe their values, to be able to articulate them or be able to 'sell' them to others. To have them and live by them is generally enough, so that the dominant communication path may be a non-verbal one. In a very real sense, for congruent leaders actions do often speak louder than words. To be present and demonstrate their values constantly is more important than speaking about them. All too often we are asked to follow leaders who are of the 'do as I say' not the 'do as I do' variety. In a world dominated by 'fake news' and social media platforms that can so easily be manipulated, looking to a leader's actions may be the last resort of followers to genuinely know that the leader is trustworthy and consistently, persistently and determinedly being true to and driven by their values.

Ask yourself: Does this leader listen to me? Are they calm? Is their message consistent? Are they approachable, visible and trustworthy? Does what they say align with what they do? Do they do what they ask others to do?

7. **Empathetic**

Congruent leaders' actions commonly drive connections, usually with people who share their values. Empathy is commonly described as 'walking in another's shoes' but it is more than this. It is about making connections with others by being able to take another's perspective, by staying away from judging others, by recognising the emotions in others (linked to emotional intelligence) and feeling 'with' people. Empathy is the lived experience of connecting to another's values. This requires that we have a sound insight into our own values and are able to recognise, respond to and connect with others from the foundation of our own values.

Congruent leaders who stand by their values and live out those values in their actions also recognise the importance of values in the lives of others. Congruent leaders are commonly followed by people who recognise and align with the values the leader has on display. Importantly the leader/follower relationship can only be effective if the congruent leader is empathetic, open, approachable and able to listen well.

8. **Competence/knowledgeable/good decision-maker**

One of the key elements of Congruent Leadership appears to relate to the leader's ability to remain credible and competent in the provision of their work or activities. Competence or knowledge is clearly linked to the practical experience and the confidence others see in the leader's ability to deliver through their actions and it means being able to show, or to do, as well as know or teach others about practical/relevant issues in line with the work/leadership area.

These attributes are all linked to the capacity of the congruent leader to deliver on the things they do. A congruent leader who is not competent, knowledgeable or able to make effective decisions is unlikely to be seen as relevant to followers and people would have little faith or trust in their ability not just to do, but constantly, persistently or effectively deliver on the values they espouse.

Being a congruent leader relies heavily on sound general knowledge and having a good knowledge base. This can also be expanded into knowing not just about work-related areas, but about how team members function, how individuals interact and the relationships between people. Congruent leaders who understand and know the things they are responsible for and are also aware of things such as people's limitations, who interacts well together, who needs a lot of support and who doesn't. Knowing who needs time on their own and who doesn't and being aware of who needs continual prompting and back-up means that congruent leaders can be present across a wider range of issues. As a result, they may be seen as more relevant or connected to a wider spectrum of people and enhancing their approachability, visibility and communication skills.

As well as having knowledge and being competent, being able to make clear and effective decisions is also aligned with a congruent leader's attributes. Decision-making, not just in relation to their work role but with regard to a whole host of issues, may be central to the effectiveness of congruent leadership.

Decision-making implies competence and sensitivity, the application of knowledge and an alignment of the decisions with the congruent leader's values.

Allied to effective decision-making is an ability to delegate appropriately and problem solve. While some people may equate decision-making with authority or power, it may also be suggested that effective decision-making is aligned with critical thinking. Perhaps it is an expression of the critical thinking that is the end point of a congruent leaders' decision-making ability with critical decisions based on an expression of the leader's values and beliefs.

9. Empowered

Empowerment is a contentious term. Empowerment is not something that can be given, but is seen here as a power that comes from within and can be activated only by an act of will. Congruent leaders may indeed be empowered to live out their lives in accordance with their values. Doing so, as mentioned, takes considerable courage and if, as suggested here, empowerment comes from within, then congruent leaders are indeed empowered. Nelson Mandela was a congruent leader. He faced multiple personal and political obstacles, not to mention years in prison, but still he was able to put into practice his values for a fair and equal society. He was visible, worked with both sides of politics and remained calm in the face of ongoing political unrest and uncertainty, but he pressed on. He put himself (and South Africa) on the road to freedom. It was, in his words 'a long walk', and this is the point. Walking is an act. He role modelled the way forward, he was visible in displaying his values about how he wanted people to engage with each other. Like Gandhi in India, he didn't just talk and he didn't just point towards a new future – he acted, moved and lived the future he saw, in the present, so that others could see the values Mandela and Gandhi held.

Congruent leaders in displaying their own empowerment are also in a position to support and motivate the empowerment of others. As role models for their own values they may be inadvertently (or consciously) motivating and inspiring others to also become empowered and to stand boldly by their own values.

10. Honesty (integrity/trustworthy)

Cantwell (2015) describes honesty as lying at the heart of true authentic leadership, and I agree. It also lies at the centre of Congruent Leadership and in this regard, Authentic and Congruent Leadership are aligned. Congruent leaders need to be honest with themselves and with others. Without honesty or integrity, they will not be trusted and are less likely to trust others. Honesty also sits at the heart of having our values on show, being empathetic and courageous. As Cantwell (2015, p. 36) states, he has 'no respect for leaders who play favourites or say one thing while doing another or whose ethical compass swings in whichever direction feels easy or most profitable at the time.' To a large degree, saying one thing while doing another is the antithesis of Congruent Leadership. Congruent leaders put on show the values they hold. Being honest and trustworthy are fundamental for the delivery of effective Congruent Leadership.

OTHER ATTRIBUTES

Over the years I have shared my views on Congruent Leadership theory and attributes and found considerable support for the characteristics offered. However, I have always been keen to explore others, and after many discussions to solicit further insights. I feel that, although not strongly evident as independent attributes, the following are frequently associated with a number of those offered above and are also worthy of consideration:

- *A good sense of humour* – not taking ourselves too seriously, even in the face of some very serious situations. Here is one example. A nurse in an intensive care unit while resuscitating a person for the third time in one shift, was performing CPR with a doctor. The doctor then lent across and said 'we really have to stop meeting like this'. It broke the tension, making the serious lifesaving event more human and bearable and allowed everyone to relax while working as an effective team.
- *Creativity* – being able to create new and novel ways of addressing problems and challenges.
- *Respect for self and others* – realising that we all have our own life journeys, that we each bring with us experiences and insights from our past history that make each of us unique and able to see the world and those around us from our own personal perspectives and that we should respect this.

WHAT CONGRUENT LEADERS ARE NOT!

Congruent leaders are not control freaks. Indeed, in the research that led to an understanding of Congruent Leadership, the one aspect or attribute that came up consistently as an attribute least looked for, or least respected in congruent leaders was 'control'. In every professional group that took part in the studies, they consistently ranked 'control' as the attribute that was least associated with congruent leadership. If the leader had any element of power or authority over the people they were leading, it was highly likely that they were not well regarded for their ability to show their values. Being in a position of control made it difficult to establish a match between the leaders' and followers' values, and the styles of communication, levels of trust and honesty, approachability and being visible were all seen to diminish as the leaders' control over the followers increased. Organisations and businesses still need to be able to exercise control over their processes and systems and, to a degree, their staff.

However, leaders who operate at the level of a translation of the organisations' values into action are less likely to require control because they lead by virtue of what they do. It is this that infuses motivation or inspiration and provides the leadership needed. Leaders cannot 'command' others to hold the values they do. This is despotism and while this will produce potentially compliant followers and power-ful leaders, it will rarely result in a happy workplace or organisation. It will rarely be profitable, it will limit people's ability to contribute new ideas and be genuinely involved in their work or role and it is not sustainable.

ACTIVITY 3.2   REFLECTIVE EXERCISE

Can you think of any other attributes that you might identify with a congruent leader? Do you have any colleagues that might fit the attributes described above? Do you fit these attributes? If you describe these attributes and the theory of Congruent Leadership to a colleague might they see you as a congruent leader?

Why not ask them?

EXAMPLES OF CONGRUENT LEADERS

Congruent Leadership is an approach to leadership that, as stated, is suitable in some circumstances and may not be as valuable or applicable as a leadership strat-egy in others. Therefore it is possible to identify leaders who could be seen as congruent leaders at some times and not at others. Winston Churchill (Britain's leader in the Second World War), for example, when holding England in virtual isolation and away from surrender after the Dunkirk evacuation and prior to the start of the Battle of Britain, could be described as a congruent leader. He showed tremendous courage in the face of significant opposition. He was visible in person and through the medium of the hour, radio. He was empathetic, being aware of the sacrifice and risk his stance would impose on the British people. He was honest with people about the risks and about his beliefs and confidence in their prospects. He was inspirational, motivational and highly charismatic. He communicated well and displayed personal empowerment to sustain his values so that he was seen as persistent, determined, dynamic and energetic. He used his vast prior experience and knowledge to help make key decisions promptly and while he may not have been the most approachable of leaders, he at least made the effort to inspire and motivate people by sharing in their suffering and risks. When Britain needed a leader who would not just point the way to victory but stand with his nation and act out the values he believed were worthy of fighting for, he became a powerful and successful leader where others in his place had struggled.

At other times and in other contexts Churchill was more dictatorial or authori-tarian. He remained determined, persistent, energetic and dynamic, but he also badgered, bothered and bullied his way to the outcomes he wanted. Given the resource constraints and stress of the war, it is not surprising that other leadership attributes sprang forth. However, at the core of his motivation in the early years of the war was a powerful connection to the values of democracy and the rights of the British people to remain independent and free from Hitler's oppression.

Abraham Lincoln (American President during the American Civil War 1861–5) is another leader who was faced with a conflict that threatened his values. Lincoln came to power just as the United States was falling apart. His fervent belief was that the United States or 'Union' needed to be preserved. This sprang from a passionate belief that the principles of democracy would not survive if the country where these principles had been established fell apart. The issue of slavery was the axe that was cutting the Union apart and he recognised that this needed to be addressed, but his primary motivation was to save the democratic principles of the United States. The American Civil War was a test of whether the founding fathers of American independence had got it right or wrong. As Guelzo (2013, p. 480) states, 'whether a democracy built solely out of the fragile reeds of constitutional propositions was merely a fuzzy pipe dream or whether people really could survive without crowns and saddles', in Lincoln's words, 'whether that nation, or any nation so conceived, and so dedicated, can long endure.' This is from Lincoln's Gettysburg address. In it he did not speak of war as a crusade for the liberation of slaves. At the beginning of the American Civil War Lincoln told his personal secretary, John Hay, that the war was necessary for 'proving that popular government is not an absurdity', for 'if we fail, it will go far to prove the incapability of the people to govern themselves.' Here Lincoln was stating his values. Slavery would fall as long as the 'Union' did not. His objective was to save the Union. Ending slavery was a necessary consequence of this objective.

In his address, made in 1864 after the consecration ceremony at Gettysburg, Lincoln made it clear that it was not what they said that day that would matter, but what those that remained did. 'The world will little note, nor long remember what we say here: while it can never forget what they did here. It is for us, the living, rather, to be dedicated here to the unfinished work which they who fought here, have thus far so nobly advanced.' This is a key aspect of Congruent Leadership. The actions of the leader matter. While this was a speech, Lincoln was reminding the 15,000 people listening that values needed to be lived in action. He reminded his audience: 'It is rather for us to be dedicated to the great task remaining before us' (to win the war and pursue it to its successful end) 'that cause for which they here gave their last full measure of devotion.'

Lincoln, like Churchill, was energetic, passionate, determined and persistent (Distinti, 2011). He was perhaps not as charismatic as other leaders, but he was able to motivate and inspire both with his actions and speeches. He was a very involved Commander in Chief, reading military theory texts to ensure he could offer sound advice to his generals, ensuring that he could become knowledgeable and competent in military matters. In each speech and in his actions, Lincoln was clear about his values. As the American Civil War came to an end, he was insistent that the way forward was a path of reconciliation, a set of values and principles that dealt fairly and gently with the Southern states as they were embraced back into the Union. In his plans for bringing the Southern or 'Rebel' states back into the Union he spoke of and practised tolerance, forgiveness and nation-building principles. Throughout his presidency he was a visible leader, in Washington, about the many Northern states and at the battlefront. He was very empathetic, frequently writing to families and mothers whose sons had been killed in action and he often issued personal pardons from execution for runaway soldiers – he even released a captured spy on the last day of the war. Lincoln was approachable and kind to White House staff and military personnel – too kind perhaps, as he had allowed his personal body guard to rest and watch the play *Our American Cousin* on the evening of his assassination. However, Lincoln died as he had lived, true to his values and courageously fighting for the unification of America and the prosperity of the United States.

In more contemporary terms, the achievements and contribution of Professor Fiona Wood, based in Western Australia, also point to a congruent leader who has dedicated her life and work to making care, specifically for burns patients, better. Through a lifetime of research and commitment to innovation she has used her values and principles to govern a congruent approach to healthcare. Part of this has laid the groundwork for a living legacy as 'Australia's Most Trusted Person' (voted for six successive years 2005–10) and as an Australian Living Treasure.

CHAPTER SUMMARY

Congruent leaders are identifiable because of where they stand and how they behave when dealing with workmates, friends and colleagues. When facing challenges in their lives they are recognisable because they display their values, beliefs and principles. They respond to challenges with consistency and courage, they are passionate, positive, determined, dynamic and energetic doers. They role model their values by being honest, visible, 'hands on' and present. They communicate well and employ empathy in their relationships with others. They are competent, knowledgeable and good at making decisions and commonly they are easy to approach, open, honest, and trustworthy. They can inspire or motivate others and may be seen as charismatic as they live out their values in the actions of their work or personal life.

Congruent leaders stand apart from novice leaders and poor decision-makers, people who lead from behind and leaders or managers who are tied up with functions focused on control, administration and structures. They may be experts in their work or professional field but are recognised, not necessarily because of their expert practice or work habits, but because when faced with challenges and critical problems their actions are directed, and their leadership is defined by the values and beliefs they hold and their respect for others.

4

VISION VERSUS VALUES

'There exists a great chasm between those, on one side, who relate everything to a single central vision ... and on the other side, those who pursue many ends, often unrelated and even contradictory ... The first kind of intellectual and artistic personality belongs to the hedgehogs, the second to the foxes.'

Isaiah Berlin; attributed to Archilochus in the *Hedgehog and the Fox* (1953)

INTRODUCTION

This chapter explores the differences in leadership theories when they are driven by different primary areas of focus. In the case of transformational leadership, the primary driver is the leader's vision; with Congruent Leadership it is the leader's values that drive them. This chapter will outline why this shift in focus matters and why the lack of a clear values-based leadership theory has led to some misrepresentation of transformational leadership, and why correcting this misconception may help leaders build stronger connections and influence through leadership that may lead to change. The chapter concludes by exploring other examples of congruent leaders.

WHAT DRIVES US MATTERS

I once spent time working as a volunteer midwifery educator at a small hospital in a rural area of Zimbabwe. I taught five groups of between 12 and 15 student midwives every six months for two and a half years and was the sole educator for the course. I taught in a classroom for a few weeks at a time and then supervised the student midwives with their practice in the labour ward, the ante-natal clinic, on the post-natal ward, in the community and in the small nursery area.

Early on, I identified that it was not uncommon for the student midwives and other qualified midwives to hit women in the labour ward. The hitting constituted slaps and flat hand hits usually to the thighs or lower legs. This was not consistent with my understanding of the management of labour and against my values. However, I needed to understand the practice before I could change it. I soon realised that part of the reason for the behaviour was that the pregnant women had very little ante-natal preparation and often came considerably under prepared for the birth. As a result, in their pain and confusion during labour the slaps were being used to focus the women on what the midwives were instructing. However, I still felt it wasn't right and I couldn't support the practice.

If I had gone in and said, 'The slapping must stop. I have a vision for how we will care for these women more effectively,' it simply would not have worked. I may well have been met with 'Who does he think he is coming to our country and telling us what to do?' Instead, I was lucky that I took a more congruent approach, without even realising it, and in so doing I put my values into action for others to see.

My approach was to role model more effective ways of preparing women early on in their labour to listen to the instructions of the student midwives. I made it clear that I would not tolerate this practice. It was something that I had never practised myself or seen anywhere else before. In this regard, I was trying to lead by example and instruct with my values to the fore, and I was successful as a leader because others saw my values on show. I was driven to instruct and role model excellent midwifery care and I was careful that my behaviour supported and matched my actions. I didn't do this consciously in the sense of having an understanding of Congruent Leadership back then. However, on reflection it is clear that a congruence of sorts formed the basis for my success in ultimately changing the practice of slapping women during labour. My motivation was not explicitly to change the practice (although I did want the hitting practice to stop), but to role model my values about respect for the women and students and quality midwifery care.

To a large extent I recognised that my leadership and role modelling brought about 'cultural change' because I used my values to highlight the contradiction between espoused culture and culture in practice. Although change resulted, I did not see myself as a transformational leader, because although it was my aim to affect and change the culture of practice, I didn't consciously set out with this aim. The students were informed that 'slapping mothers' was not appropriate. However, it was my ability to role model the desired behaviour that led to the change. Students said they were influenced by watching me practice in the labour ward. One said, my 'enthusiasm for the welfare of the woman made her want to do better.' Another said, my 'presence in the labour ward, talking quietly and showing I cared for the women created in her a desire for instructing the women without hitting them.' My hope was to improve care and stop the midwife's practice of hitting the women and I did so by focusing on my own values and supporting the students to become aware of their own, as I role modelled another way to behave.

I did not provide an 'idealised influence' or 'inspirational motivation' (Vaismoradi et al., 2016, p. 975). I simply did what I thought was the right thing to do, consistently. I didn't have a vision for how I would change the behaviour or practice – indeed I was a guest in another culture and I was careful not to make changing anything my aim. Instead, I was respectful, avoided an attitude of control and began by talking calmly and patiently with the pregnant women and student midwives. I did what I thought was right and based my actions on appropriate midwifery practice.

Without realising it, and years before I started to explore and understand Congruent Leadership, I had stumbled upon an approach to leadership that was very much driven by and based upon my values. Congruent Leadership, it would seem, may be a fair fit to describe the approach I had taken in that labour ward in Zimbabwe.

Leaders who are focused upon transforming practice or their workplace may sometimes fall into the trap of using control and power, authority and deadlines to force change. Even with the best intentions in the world, this is seldom the best way to bring about change. If vision is the driver, the risk may be that sometimes the end (ironically) blinds us to the cost of the change being imposed.

In another example of what drives us matters, I offer the sinking of the *Titanic* in 1912. The owner of the ship, Mr Joseph Ismay of the White Star Line (who was on board for the maiden voyage), valued speed and his company's reputation for luxury and service. It was these values that drove the company and dominated their approach to their business and their clients/customers. Safety was less prominent in their considerations and, as such, the captain was ordered to advance, full steam ahead, into an area known to contain an ice field. It is perhaps true that the builders and owners were overconfident in their ship, but had they been driven to value safety over speed, the outcome for the *Titanic* and the people on board may have been very different.

VISION

Vision is the focus of transformational leadership. This theory was developed as an attempt to understand the distinction between leadership and management (Downton, 1973; Bass, 1985; Bennis and Nanus, 1985; Northouse, 2016) and to consider the question of why some leaders are able to inspire their followers even when the situation is less than ideal. House (1976) and Burns (1978) secured the term's distinction by making the link between the leader and followers' motives. The theory was then refined to support a link between the leaders' vision and the motivation of the followers. Followers then looked to the leader for an idealised influence or inspirational motivation from the leader's vision.

Transformational leadership is about challenging the status quo by creating a vision and sharing that vision. In this way, successful transformational leaders are able to establish and gain support for their vision while being driven towards maintaining momentum and empowerment. The word and application of 'vision' is central to the theory of transformational leadership. In addition to vision, there is also a connection to an 'idealised influence' and 'inspirational motivation' as followers recognise and become inspired or motivated. The leader, who is commonly trusted, has self-confidence or self-knowledge and can communicate well, sets out the plan of their vision and the followers are motivated to follow this leader (over others who may be less articulate, less trustworthy or have less confidence to be able to deliver on their vision).

The interdependence of followers and leaders within transformational leadership theory has meant that it has found favour in a wide range of industries, institutions, businesses and organisations. Transformational leadership really does have a place in the spectrum of leadership theories that leaders can access to effect change and build support for people within an organisation. As well as being a foundation for the leader's vision, transformational leadership is significant because it is related to the establishment to change. It is this link that has really bolstered the desire to secure the place of transformational leadership in the healthcare and educational domains, as well as a range of other businesses and industries.

Where leaders are required to or wish to establish a vision and create the drive to inspire or motivate their colleagues, transformational leadership should be fostered and developed. However, the dominance of a transformational leadership model in a number of industries, institutions and business areas, with its focus on leaders who are 'visionary' and with an assumption that leadership and status go hand in hand, has meant that different perspectives of leadership have not been widely developed or accepted.

Many industries, institutions, businesses and organisations have looked for, and to, leaders with their eye on the horizon, leaders who were politically and managerially aware, 'visionaries' who could take their professions, industries or businesses forward and who were able to inspire and motivate their employees, teams or colleagues with their vision. As such, transformational leaders are commonly in positions of authority or power, where not only can they initiate change, they can push it through.

However, I suspect transformational leadership has been manipulated to fit a desired outcome without a full recognition of the type of leadership that was taking place, or what was really happening from a follower perspective. This is not a criticism, but an observation based on the realisation of this effect over years of research in the leadership domain. It may be that in describing types of leadership we commonly refer to familiar reference points and prior knowledge to make current theories fit, rather than find new ways to explain what was observed or occurred.

MAKING THEORIES FIT

I did this myself during the pilot study of my doctoral thesis looking at nursing leadership. I tried to use transformational leadership theory to explain the pilot study results and was sure that transformational leadership would be the best fit to describe the leaders who were identified. However, as more and more of the general study results came back they pointed to a lack of focus on 'vision' in the respondent's comments and I was left to wonder if indeed the theory and the phenomenon I was seeing complemented each other at all. Transformational leadership theory was what I had anticipated finding because, at the time, this was the best theory to fit the field of practice and study I was involved with. However, at the time I was not looking for a new theory and made do with an established theory to explain the outcomes and results I observed. In fact, in some cases established theories are moulded to accommodate the results researchers seek. This is not a criticism of other researchers or their work, but a simple appreciation that sometimes we use what we know as a reference point for what we see or hope to see.

Here is another example in a study by Vaismoradi et al. (2016). They describe the actions of a number of nurse educators as 'transformational' because they changed students' practice by outlining their vision. Yet in the article they rarely refer to the educator's vision but focus very firmly on their ability and desire to inspire and motivate their followers and offer an idealised influence. The influence was offered in each case through role modelling of their values and beliefs about providing exceptional care and safe medication practices. In effect they were doing what Day et al. (2000, p. 15) described as 'purposefully impact[ing] upon the culture in order to change it.' However, the educators described in the medication safety article (Vaismoradi et al., 2016) affected the culture and practice not because they laid out their vision (even though goals were mentioned), but because they led and influenced others by role modelling, instructing and practising in accord with the values and beliefs that supported exceptional and safe practice. In effect they were being congruent leaders.

From an organisational perspective it is also worth noting that vision relates to where an organisation is going and what it is doing. Values are about how an organisation goes about what it is doing. Values drive decisions and become the foundation of the culture, contributing to the design and function of the operating system and organisational structure (Stanley, 2017). In this light, a values-based culture underpins the organisation's vision and if the values and beliefs also link to people's emotional and relationship networks, congruent leaders are in a position to influence and build powerful and lasting organisational change and culture.

In the questionnaire phase of my own studies, the term 'visionary' was identified by a significant number of respondents as being affiliated with leadership, although even when mentioned strongly, it appeared only as the 27th ranked word on a list of 42 words to describe the qualities and characteristics most associated with leadership, bringing into question the significance of 'visionary' as a quality or characteristic sought or seen in some aspects of leadership. In addition, research respondents were invited to list their own attributes of leaders and as such identified an additional 85 characteristics, with only three relating to 'vision', 'being visionary' or 'being forward thinking' (Stanley, 2006a, 2006b).

The lack of characteristics centred around shopfloor, coalface or bedside leaders being visionary was borne out by the results of the interviews, where 'vision' was hardly mentioned as an attribute looked for in this type of leader and rarely described as the motivation behind being this type of leader.

VALUES

In the business world O'Reilly and Pfeffer (2000) and Gentile (2010) see values as crucial. In comparing the performance of a number of companies with superior results in their area of speciality, the more successful companies had an approach to leadership that was based on values. Values, they felt, came first and acted as guiding principles that helped these companies to make crucial and difficult decisions. O'Reilly and Pfeffer (2000) also noted that the values these successful companies held were not prioritised as such, but that the companies operated in such a way that their values were enacted and they worked hard to resolve clashes of values. Focusing on values meant that the businesses were able to build trust, motivation and commitment (O'Reilly and Pfeffer, 2000).

Hall (2005) supports this view suggesting that companies who addressed and followed sound ethical practices were much more likely to be profitable and successful – by a considerable margin. Kouzes and Posner (2010) offered similar research in which they demonstrated that employees in organisations where they are clear about the organisations' values and also had high clarity about their own personal values had a greater commitment to the organisation. Significantly, it was a correlation between a person's own values and a match with the organisations' values that drew the strongest commitment. Their conclusion was that people cannot commit fully to anything unless it fits with their own beliefs or values (Kouzes and Posner, 2010). This is a powerful concept for employees and employers to grasp because many people enter their career, profession or employment because they want to make a difference and because they want to work with people and help make a difference for or with others.

WHAT IS MEANT BY VALUES?

What is meant by values? Values can be described as deeply held views that act as guiding principles for individuals and organisations (Pendleton and King, 2002). They are different to ethics which suggest a system of rules or standards to which people are expected to comply or apply (Gentile, 2010). Values, however, are about something we own ourselves – *my values*, or *your values* or something we agree on collectively, *our values*. They are things we experience or hold onto deeply, they are things we feel and engage in thinking about, although they may not even register on a cognitive level, unless promoted. They are not morals, which rest upon an understanding of what we understand to be 'right' and 'wrong' conduct. Values are about something with an inherent worth or quality to us or our society. Values can be an object or an idea, a thing or a stance. These types of values may have a moral or ethical aspect to them and are akin to virtues. Our values can be individual, communal, societal, family-centric, ethnically based, culturally guided, built around our personal experiences, educational and religious influences, professional and employment experiences and, in more recent times, guided or motivated by electronic media, TV, cinema, the internet, social media and other forms of communication. As such, all these terms are interrelated and Congruent Leadership is very much focused on values-based leadership and how people lead from an understanding of their values.

RECOGNISING VALUES

In the research undertaken to support the development of Congruent Leadership theory, respondents from a range of health professional disciplines stated and made explicit that it was their values that were central to the development of trust. They watched the way people behaved to determine their values and it was this that bolstered their followership. It was this link that formed the basis of trust in their follower/leader relationship and if values were stated and not consistently shown, trust was harmed. Values were also seen to relate to where individuals or organisations stand on a range of social issues and pointed toward actions or statements that reflected what was important to that person or organisation.

When applied to understanding this type of leadership, Antrobus and Kitson (1999, p. 750) identified 'understanding self and having a clear understanding of values, purpose and personal meaning' as part of the skills repertoire they identified for leaders. Being creative and having a vision remains central to the successful application of transformational leadership (Frankel, 2008), although this appears not to be a feature for which congruent leaders are recognised (Stanley, 2008, 2011, 2017). There is a view that values are inextricably linked to vision, although Pendleton and King (2002) declare that it may be even more important to know where you stand (a values-centred position) rather than where you are going (pertaining to vision), implying that values are rooted in understanding an individual's and an organisation's principles, while vision is about being able to drive through or respond to changes in the future. Vision and values are linked. They are not in direct opposition and in many cases values form the basis on which vision may rest. However, they do offer different drivers for what might motivate a leader or point to how a leader may be perceived.

Two questions emerge: 'What are our values?' 'What might leadership that is based on values look like?' The second question is the point of this book. In response to the first question ... I was recently asked what my professional values might be. I had been interested in this myself and have spent many years seeking an answer. As such, I have asked thousands of nursing students (as they embark on their nursing career journey) and qualified nurses (engaged in the study of clinical leadership) to describe what they saw as the key or most significant values of their professional group (nursing). While more an ad hoc set of enquiries than a research project, it may come as no surprise that the following ten are offered most consistently. In the UK, the Chief Nurse of the National Health Service (NHS) in the UK established a set of six key values that go some way to establishing a core set of values for health professionals in the NHS (DoH, 2013; NHS England, 2013). They are shown in comparison to the list of ten core nursing values I have identified below (see Table 4.1).

Table 4.1   Top ten health professional values/UK Chief Nurse's 6 Cs

Health professional values	UK Chief Nurse's 6 Cs
• Honesty/truthfulness/integrity • Trustworthiness • Compassion/care • Respect • Reliability • Clinical knowledge • Organised • Communication skills • Professionalism • Fairness	• Compassion • Care • Clinical knowledge • Clear interpersonal skills • Communication skills • Courage

Others that get a mention but are not as constantly cited are: listening/competence/creativity/self-control and humility.

Source: DoH (2013).

In the leadership research studies described in Chapter 2, 'vision' or 'being visionary' was seldom cited as an attribute of grassroots, shopfloor, bedside or coalface leaders (Stanley, 2006a, 2006b, 2008, 2011, 2017). Significantly the results from these studies also suggested that these types of leaders are evident at all levels of an organisation (or business) and may not be tagged to formal positions of authority or power. As such, these types of leaders were seen at all levels of an organisation, although many were not aware that they were identified as leaders. This type of leader is commonly nominated or identified as such because of their passion for their job, their commitment to the core competencies of the role (or their colleagues' needs), their skills and knowledge or their engagement with their work. It was only rarely their ability to articulate a vision that singled them out as leaders. They were seen as inspirational and motivational, enthusiastic and strongly connected to the process of addressing the needs of followers (even if they didn't know they had any). These attributes could be attributed to transformational leadership, except that the central feature of it – vision – is missing.

These leaders appeared at odds with the principal aspects of transformational leadership where the transformational leader possessed a vision of some future state

(Bass, 1985, 1990). The links to an idealised influence, inspirational motivation, were evident but less well defined and the influence was more likely to be based on 'real-world' actions and practice. Inspiration and motivation were evident but were also based on the values and beliefs of the leader as translated through their actions or work practices. It was not a case of 'being optimistic about the future' or 'aspiring to excellence' (Vaismoradi et al., 2016, p. 975). It was about living and practising in the now and demonstrating excellence in the current workplace environment.

VALUES NOW!

The leaders identified in the research studies that underpin this text didn't aspire to excellence in the future. They didn't say, 'I have a vision for how I will care for these patients today ...' They didn't appear at the roadside accident and say 'Wait ... I have a vision for the management of this RTA ...' They didn't appear in a physiotherapy clinic and say, 'I see a clinic with more space and greater patient flow patterns ...' These leaders may have had ideas about improving their service and making change happen, but the leaders I encountered in the research were principally recognised by their followers because they did what was needed to the best of their abilities, in keeping with best practice, and in so doing led others with their values on show and with their beliefs to the fore.

Tracey Chapman said it best in a song from her debut album *Tracey Chapman* in 1987. In this one line she was able to indicate that something promised for the future is of no value, if the values of the person in the present are not expressed. Values matter over vision.

'A love declared for days to come is as good as none.'

(Song) Tracey Chapman.

Values are related to now, about actions now, about the application of values in the present, and if they are not evident in the present, they are of little value if declared for the future. Values are only of value if they are acted upon, evident in what we do and able to be recognised. Values without actions are just rhetoric and many a politician has been caught out offering to describe their values for the future while doing the opposite in the present or never following up on their promises. The net result of this is still a statement of the politician's values, but it is not a stance or value set that is recognised as consistent with what was promised. As such, you cannot not be displaying your values. Vision-based leadership is forward-looking and centred on goals, aims, plans, hopes and aspirations ... not on the now, not on the present. Leaders with the vision are vital and needed, but we also need to recognise the significance of leaders who live on the path of their values.

Congruent Leadership is values and actions focused. Congruent leaders can be anyone across the organisation but in each case they apply their values in action and as such their values have no meaning unless they are visible: actions of the now. Making tomorrow better means acting on and recognising appropriate values today.

It is proposed that while transformational leadership has a powerful place in supporting leaders with the specific goal of bringing about change and who are commonly in positions of hierarchical power or have senior roles and responsibilities to drive change. There remains a gap between the characteristics of a Transformational Leadership and alternative theories such as 'Breakthrough Leadership' (Sarros and Butchatsky, 1996), 'Authentic Leadership' (Bhindi and Duignan, 1997; George, 2003; Cantwell, 2015) and Congruent Leadership (Stanley, 2008, 2011, 2017) and the reality of leading on the shopfloor, at the bedside or in any location or level. Congruent Leadership explains why leaders who do not exercise control or power are followed. It is because their values and beliefs stem from and match their actions. For an elaboration of the key features of both Congruent Leadership and transformational leadership (see Table 4.2).

Table 4.2   A comparison of the features of Transformational and Congruent Leadership

Transformational Leadership	Congruent Leadership
• Establishing direction • Aligning people • **Motivating and inspiring** • Produces change – often dramatic • About where you are going (vision) • **Effective communicators** • Creative/initiative	• **Motivating and inspiring** • Approachable/open • Actions based on values and beliefs • About where you stand (principles) • **Effective communicators** • Visible • Empowered
Recognised leadership/management, hierarchical or titled positions.	*Any level, not necessary to have a title or hierarchical position* *Guided by passion, compassion* *Build enduring relationships*

Note: Although there are some similarities (in bold) the key differences relate to what motivates the leaders: vision or values and principles.

EXAMPLES OF CONGRUENT LEADERS

Not all congruent leaders are political or military leaders. Mary Seacole – 'Mother Seacole' – was born Mary Jane Grant in Kingston, Jamaica, in 1805. She had a mixed-race (free Creole) mother and a Scottish-born, officer father. Her mother ran a boarding house for sick and injured soldiers and sailors and it was here that Mary began to learn her medical and nursing skills. Mary's mother was a noted 'doctress' who used traditional Caribbean and African herbal remedies to heal and tend the sick in her care. Mary grew up enjoying relative freedom at a time in Jamaica where to be black implied a slave ancestry or connections to slavery. Creoles though were still restricted in what they could do and Mary could not join a profession, hold public office or exercise extensive civil rights, although she was far more fortunate than the majority of slaves that dominated the island.

Mary received a sound education and further developed her medical knowledge. In 1821 she travelled to London for the first time. When she returned to Jamaica she continued to learn much from her mother and also travelled about the Caribbean and parts of Central America where she learnt more about medicine and disease.

Mary's husband Edwin Horatio Hamilton Seacole (rumoured to be an illegitimate son of Horatio Nelson and Emma, Lady Hamilton) died in 1844, and after a time of deep grief, Mary turned a 'bold front to fortune' and assumed the management of her mother's hotel. She threw herself into her work, declining many offers of marriage. In 1850 she treated patients suffering from a cholera epidemic that killed an estimated 32,000 Jamaicans. Mary, with great insight into the transmission of disease, recognised that the outbreak of the epidemic was likely to be attributed to a steamship that had arrived from New Orleans, Louisiana. Her experience in dealing with cholera was to prove vital later in her life.

In 1851 she travelled to Panama, Central America and arrived in time to treat the first victim of a cholera outbreak there. The patient survived and Mary's reputation as a healer was cemented. Other patients came to her for care and while the rich paid, she treated the poor for free. Many people died, but her willingness and commitment to confront the disease and persist in finding a cure ensured she was held in high regard. In 1853 she returned to Jamaica and was immediately recruited by the medical authorities to help deal with an outbreak of yellow fever. Mary's response was to recruit a number of other Afro-Caribbean women and set up a hospital outside Kingston where they cared for people who suffered from the disease. Following the subsidence of the outbreak, Mary learned about the escalating conflict in the Crimea and she decided to volunteer and set off to enlist as a nurse in London.

Mary was unable to convince the British medical or military authorities to use her. Even though the Nightingale nurses that travelled to the Crimean War were understaffed, Mary, due to her skin colour, was refused an interview or an opportunity to go with the Nightingale nurses. Not to be put off Mary applied to the publicly subscribed Crimean Fund to travel independently but was again refused. Undaunted, Mary raised her own funds with the help of a doctor from Panama and set off for the Crimea. On the way she stopped at Malta and a doctor returning from the Crimea wrote a letter of recommendation and introduction to Florence Nightingale for Mary to use on her arrival. On arriving in Constantinople Mary arranged to travel across the Bosporus to Scutari but was unsuccessful in securing a place with the 'Nightingale' nurses.

Mary, having come this far, transferred her supplies to another ship and set off for the seat of the fighting on the Crimean Peninsula, arriving at Balaclava early in 1855. There she built a 'hotel' at a place called Spring Hill. The 'hotel' was built from driftwood, packing cases, iron sheets and house parts scavenged from the nearby town of Kamara. She used local labour and opened the newly christened 'British Hotel' in March 1855. The 'hospital' opened six days a week providing provisions and food for French and British soldiers. It was little more than a collection of huts, one of which served as a small hospital ward. Mary provided tea and coffee and dealt with medical complaints in the mornings and then set off to visit casualties about the battlefields in the afternoons.

Mary made a point of visiting the battlefields and treating wounded and ill men often under fire. On one occasion she dislocated her right thumb while in the trenches, an injury which never completely healed. A *Times* newspaper special correspondent said of Mary that she was a 'warm and successful physician, who doctors and cures for all manner of men with extraordinary success. She is always in attendance near the battle-field to aid the wounded and has earned many a poor fellow's blessing.' A soldier said of Mary, 'she had the secret of a recipe for cholera and dysentery, and liberally dispensed the specific, alike to those who could pay and those who could not. It was bestowed with an amount of personal kindness which, though not an item of the original prescription, she deemed essential to the cure.'

So closely involved in the front-line care of soldiers was Mary that she was the first woman into Sevastopol (Sebastopol) after the siege was lifted. The war's conclusion brought ruin as the trade at the British Hotel diminished and Mary returned to England poorer than she had left. Soon Mary was declared bankrupt. However, the Seacole Testimonial Fund was established to offer support. In July 1857 the Seacole Fund Grand Military Festival was held to contribute to her Testimonial Fund. The event was supported by many military men and over a thousand artists performed including eleven military bands with an attendance of over 40,000. Mary also produced an autobiography, *The Wonderful Adventures of Mrs. Seacole in Many Lands*, the first book written by a black woman in Britain. Gradually Mary regained her financial footing and when she died in 1881, in London, she was once more financially independent.

Mary Seacole's many achievements in the Crimean War were somewhat overshadowed by Florence Nightingale's fame and while well known in her lifetime she has since faded (a little) from the pages of history. She is famous in the Caribbean, and there has been a resurgence of interest in her contribution to nursing in recent years. In 2004, Mary was voted into first place in an online poll of 100 Great Black Britons and her contribution to nursing and medical care in Central America, the Caribbean and the Crimean solidify her place as a supreme clinically focused leader.

The story of Mary Seacole is offered as another example of a congruent leader. She was empowered, courageous, driven by her values, passionate about helping others, persistent, determined, dynamic and energetic. She was open, approachable and trusted. She was visible on the battlefield and in the service of people with contagious diseases. She displayed great empathy as she demonstrated her knowledge and competence in tropical diseases and wound management. She set out to work with others and even after numerous rejections took it upon herself to travel to the seat of the fighting and invest herself in what she thought was an important role. Mary decided to go to the Crimea at the risk of her life, reputation and financial security – she did what she believed was the right thing to do.

On 5 June 1989, a single man dressed in a white shirt and black trousers stood defiantly before a long line of Red Army tanks as they attempted to leave Tiananmen Square in Beijing. As the tanks turned to avoid him he stepped into their path. They turned back, again to avoid him, but he stepped back into their path again. He stood his ground, until eventually the tank's engines were turned off. The man then climbed up on the first tank and spoke to the commander. Although no one knows exactly what he said, it is reported that he chastised the tank commander for taking part in the brutal suppression (slaughter) of the protesters in Tiananmen Square.

His name is not known, nor is his fate, because at the end of the standoff he was grabbed by two men and disappeared into the crowd that had gathered to watch. We will never know if these men were friends taking him to safety or goons taking him to a prison, or worse. What is remarkable about this event is that although the student uprising that was a catalyst to his protest failed, the image of 'tank man' (captured on film and broadcast around the world) as he stood courageously before a line of lethal armour, symbolises the raw heroism of an ordinary person and offers another example of a congruent leader in action.

Here was a man, not a great politician, not a military leader and not a person with titled leadership responsibility, standing (literally) for what he believed in. He didn't look on or shout his disapproval from the wings. He stood up, walked out and held his ground. He was not seeking to voice a vision or to take control and we don't even know his name. Yet *Time Magazine* named him one of the 100 most influential people of the twentieth century. His influence, his leadership, came from the expression of his beliefs and values in action. He courageously sought to defy the tanks and make a point about their inhumanity, but he didn't seek to express a vision for a future state. The image of him standing resolutely before the tanks in Tiananmen Square has impacted on global consciousness and China's domestic and international policy in subtle yet significant ways. 'Tank man' offers another example of a congruent leader.

CHAPTER SUMMARY

My initial exploration of leadership looked for a match between the bedside, coalface, shopfloor leaders' practice and transformational leadership. I had begun with a hypothesis where I imagined that this type of leader would fit the description of transformational leadership theory (Stanley, 2004). I thought they would be seen as enthusiastic, motivated, creative and visionary or described as having elaborate visions of where they wanted their followers to go and that their colleagues, inspired by their idealised leadership and descriptions of their vision, goals or plans, would be willing followers.

The results from my initial research challenged these preconceptions. My initial research confirmed that while these types of leaders were seen as motivational and enthusiastic, they were not followed or recognised because of their vision. This was confirmed with each subsequent study, and as the studies were completed with different professional groups in different countries with different gender mixes over a period of many years and with various methodologies, they confirmed that transformational leadership did not suit or explain why bedside, coalface or shopfloor leaders were seen as such. It was soon clear that another theory of leadership based on values was needed. It was evident that some leaders were followed because their actions were embedded in their values and beliefs and these resonated with their followers. Congruent Leadership seems to fit the bill of a theory that supports this type of, and focus on, leadership.

Congruent Leadership theory was developed (or was discovered) in an attempt to fill the gap in an understanding of non-hierarchical, non-authoritarian or non-power-based leadership and shed light on why some leaders, without formal power or a big office, are able to lead or become recognised as leaders. It is suggested here that followers are drawn to or identify with leaders who can lead them through the 'here and now' issues of sometimes busy and chaotic work environments. These are leaders who can cope with the demands of each day as it comes, rather than postulate and pontificate about how things could or should be. Congruent leaders are seen and selected when they have their values on show and stand on a foundation built or linked directly to their values. Congruent Leadership, therefore, is defined in action, as leaders mobilise their values and beliefs to guide and direct what they do when faced with the challenges and critical problems of their life, workplace or social world (Clark, 2008; Stanley, 2008, 2011, 2017).

5

THE STRENGTHS AND
LIMITATIONS OF
CONGRUENT LEADERSHIP

'Find people who share your values, and you'll conquer the world together.'

John Ratzenberger, American actor

INTRODUCTION

This chapter outlines the strengths and the limitations of Congruent Leadership theory. There are always questions around theories. There always will be. This is the nature of theories ... and this is a good thing too. At the start of his book *A Brief History of Time*, Stephen Hawking (1988) discusses a range of theories for the origins of the universe and how mankind understood the earth to sit in the celestial scheme of things. Given that we don't yet know 100 per cent how the universe originated, Hawking describes his views as a theory, and rightly so, because any theory can only be a hypothesis until it is proven conclusively. Congruent Leadership theory, while based on sound research designs, sound methodologies, a number of different studies conducted over time in different countries and with different professional groups, and using sound analysis of the data, can still be questioned, and it should continue to be tested and examined. As such it remains a theory.

This chapter outlines arguments in support of, and against, the hypothesis for Congruent Leadership theory. As with the two previous chapters, this chapter concludes by exploring examples of congruent leaders.

THE STRENGTHS OF CONGRUENT LEADERSHIP

There are a number of strengths afforded by understanding and applying Congruent Leadership. These are outlined below.

GRASSROOTS LEADERS

One of the main strengths of Congruent Leadership is that it supports the promotion of 'grassroots' leaders (Roberts, 1983, p. 29). Roberts and others have suggested that finding ways to liberate leaders within the core group, without plucking them from the rank and file of staff or employees, will ensure that leaders can develop who remain focused on the core issues, values and beliefs that are relevant to and affect the interests and work of the core group. The congruent leader's credibility is recognised and established when their actions match their values and beliefs. As such it is their ability to demonstrate or display their actions and not their position, title, authority or role that facilitates their ability to lead.

Congruent Leadership places power in the hands of anyone who is prepared to act in concert with their values and beliefs in spite of opposition, financial disadvantage, embarrassment and even loss of social and personal respect. Congruent Leadership can be exercised by anyone, at any level of an organisation and be used as a leadership theory to recognise the significance of leadership from a grassroots perspective.

An added advantage of Congruent Leadership is that leaders can be seen to be anyone from any walk of life or any level in an organisation. They can also come from any professional group or employee level even if they do not fit the mould or type of leadership commonly referred to in textbooks or theories that only recognise leaders who are chief executive officers (CEOs), generals, managers or political dynamos. In this regard Congruent Leadership supports the implementation and application of interdisciplinary practice and learning. When different health professional groups are linked by shared values about care, practice or how they relate to clients or patients, then there can be shared leadership based on a common understanding of values. As such this approach to values-based leadership is highly relevant for interprofessional, collaborative or interdisciplinary working. Team work across professional groups is then enhanced, with patient safety being more likely to be the focus of the interprofessional exchange.

Vital for health professionals is also the advantage of having a leadership theory that has a name describing this 'other' type of approach to leadership. Naming this type of leadership, which has for a long time been lost under the weight of leadership theories and conversations that have pinned leadership to management, power or authority, means these 'other' leaders will no longer be unrecognised and greater potential leadership, change and innovation will stem from their being able to recognise themselves as leaders and confidently say, 'I am a congruent leader'.

RECOGNISING THEMSELVES AS LEADERS

Congruent Leadership helps grassroots leaders at any level in a range of different health professional groups who lead on an everyday basis. It offers a name for the type of leadership approach they employ and can identify with. The realisation that there is a theory that is not just for authoritative, transactional or managerial leaders may lead to an increase in grassroots, shopfloor, factory floor, office, classroom, clinic and bedside level leaders actually seeing themselves as leaders. Many of the people interviewed in the research who support this theory offered detailed descriptions of congruent leaders but failed to recognise these qualities or attributes in themselves even when others could.

Current leadership theories that emphasise 'vision' or link leadership and management responsibilities close avenues of expression or understanding for those leaders who lead without formal authority or recognised power, without a function related to change or titles that encompass leadership. Congruent Leadership theory, based as it is on the match between the leader's actions and their values and beliefs, offers a new and liberating way of describing leaders that is not addressed in previous views of leadership or management.

FOUNDATION FOR OTHER THEORIES

Another strength of Congruent Leadership is that it offers a foundation for other theories to rest upon (see Figure 5.1). From this foundation, grassroots leaders can solidify an understanding and connection with the core values and beliefs about their work (profession, business, organisational role). From this foundation leaders are able to recognise their values and beliefs and the contribution these make to who they are and their relationship to the organisation in which they work. This foundation also helps the non-traditional leaders' acknowledgement that a recognition of their approach to leadership is as valid as any other approach or style of leadership.

A STRONG LINK BETWEEN VALUES AND ACTIONS

A significant strength of Congruent Leadership is that it builds a strong link between values, beliefs and actions. In this regard it is not static, but dynamic. Authentic leadership (Bhindi and Duignan, 1997; George, 2003), like Congruent Leadership, describes leaders who have a genuine 'desire to serve others through their leadership' (George, 2003, p. 12). Many of the attributes for both types of leadership are similar. However, Congruent Leadership makes explicit the link between purpose, meaning and values as well as the leader's commitment to acting

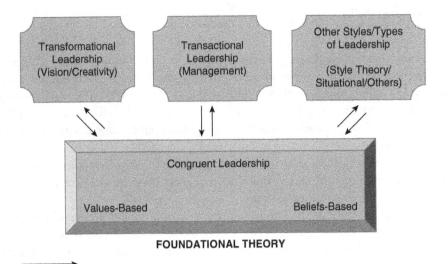

FOUNDATIONAL THEORY

→

The arrows represent the interdependence and relationships between Congruent Leadership and the adjacent theories. Congruent Leadership theory offers a foundation on which 'grassroots' leaders (and others) can build skills and insights into the other leadership theories.

Figure 5.1   **The relationship of Congruent Leadership to other leadership theories/ models**

upon them and in accordance with them. Congruence is a statement of agreement and consistency and using this word in describing the type of leadership helps promote the link between values, beliefs, meaning and actions. In effect, having beliefs and recognising one's own values and knowing where you stand is of little merit if they are not employed when faced with challenges, or if they are not displayed in or congruent with your actions.

Voicing one's values (Gentile, 2010) is also of little value if the voice is meek, unheard or removed from the context of the work or organisational application, or if expressed values are not then followed up with actions. Authors in support of authentic leadership (Bhindi and Duignan, 1997; George, 2003; Wong and Cummings, 2009, Cantwell, 2015) recognise this to some extent, with George (2003) indicating that authentic leadership is about 'being yourself, being the person you were created [*sic*] to be' (George, 2003, p. 11), although Cantwell (2015) very much links authentic leadership with actions.

However, Congruent Leadership is more than just 'being'. It is about acting, displaying, demonstrating and living the leaders' values and beliefs, even if unconsciously. Congruent Leadership although similar to authentic leadership, emphasises the translation of values and beliefs into action. Indeed, it is the act of living out one's values that prompted the recognition of Congruent Leadership. For it is only in action that leadership is evident and effective. Leaders demonstrating a congruent approach are recognised and feel valued for the contribution they make and for the value they add to the organisation, business or institution.

SUPPORTS FURTHER UNDERSTANDING OF NON-POSITIONAL, NON-HIERARCHICAL LEADERSHIP

One of the main benefits of Congruent Leadership is in advancing an understanding of leadership that is not based on positions of power, authority or senior hierarchy. Congruent Leadership supports leaders in any work environment and in all health professional groups, where leaders are not invested with authority or a title to lead. They are seen where leaders function in the trenches, at the front-line, at the coalface, on the shopfloor, on the factory floor or in direct proximity to the product delivery or service user. Recognising, promoting or developing Congruent Leadership may be of benefit. Recognising that leaders can be anyone means accepting that leadership can and does occur at any level and across all sections of an organisation, business, industry or professional group. One clear advantage of this type of leadership approach is that it may bolster leaders who have traditionally been afforded less of a voice at the development and innovation table. There are many congruent leaders, at all levels and in a range of workplace environments, and they bring with them the drive to represent the values and core principles of their work role, talents, contributions or professional skills. It is my contention that the recognition of Congruent Leadership will enhance the organisation, business or industry, foster a greater focus on a values-based approach to work and give greater voice and influence to the many people who lead without big offices, leather chairs, their name on the door or the power to hire and fire.

ANYONE CAN BE A CONGRUENT LEADER

Congruent leaders are found in a range of positions and across the spectrum of an organisation, business or industry. As such, the application of Congruent Leadership is not limited to people in leadership, titled or senior positions. Anyone can apply or demonstrate Congruent Leadership if they are encouraged and supported to see the significance of their values and beliefs applied to their work role.

In many leadership texts or theoretical descriptions of leadership the leaders are kings or queens, CEOs, have titles, positions, authority and recognised power. However, a key strength of Congruent Leadership is that it rests on the recognition of the leader's values by others, as evident in their actions. In each of the research studies described in the final chapter of this book, the leaders identified were commonly not in senior or management positions. For values to be the leader's driving force others need to see them and the leader needs to be visible or 'present'. Therefore anyone who is visible, present and prepared to demonstrate their values and beliefs could be seen by others as a leader. Joan of Arc was 12 or 14 years of age, had no power, title or authority, yet she was able to lead the French army to a series of stunning victories by putting into practice the strength of her values, and power of her beliefs (see the examples of congruent leaders below). Scenario 5.1 offers another example of how anyone can be a congruent leader.

SCENARIO 5.1   CONGRUENT LEADERSHIP IN ACTION

DUTCH SOLDIER ON THE *BATAVIA*

The story of the wreck of the *Batavia* off the coast of Western Australia at the Abrolis Islands in 1629 is one layered with tragedy and heroism (Fitzsimons, 2012): a ship-wreck in the night, a greedy, evil high-ranking official (Jeronimus Cornelisz), an absent captain and senior officer, murder, cannibalism, rape and cruelty. There is possibly one bright episode within the whole story. That is the conduct and courage of a Dutch soldier, called Wiebbe Hayes. He was noted when the shipwreck occurred helping others to safety and staying calm and focused while torment and destruction raged all about him. Later when the situation on the island became desperate it was Wiebbe who led a group of men to search for and find water so that they could help others. He was also responsible for organising the defence of their island against the evil high-ranking official. This soldier was present, visible, communicated well and shared the resources out fairly.

Wiebbe was recognised at the time as having saved many lives and for having stood up to the evil and cruel position of the men led by Jeronimus Cornelisz. He was not an officer or a well-travelled seaman, he was not in a senior position with the Dutch East India Company and yet he came to the fore and led a number of people to safety and survival. He was rewarded with a promotion, a small monetary reward and then was lost to history's records. However, it was because he stood by his val-ues and beliefs that he was able to help others to survive. This was not the result of a predetermined plan or a vision, but the act of a man who understood that to help other people get through the disaster of the shipwreck and cruelty of Jeronimus Cornelisz, he had to stand up and do what was needed.

SIGNIFICANT SUBSTANTIATION

The research that supports Congruent Leadership has been significant (Bishop, 2009a, 2009b; Stanley, 2006a, 2006b, 2006c, 2006d, 2007, 2008, 2009, 2010, 2011, 2012, 2013a, , 2014, 2017; Stanley and Sherratt, 2010; Stanley and Stanley, 2017; Stanley, Cuthbertson and Latimer, 2012; Stanley, Hutton and Atkinson, 2014; Stanley, Blanchard et al., 2017). In addition, the details of Congruent Leadership theory have been exposed to large numbers of my professional peers at conferences and before a raft of health professional students studying a range of courses in a number of countries and contexts (e.g. Thailand, Singapore, Tanzania, Canada, the UK, Ireland and Australia). The theory is being tested in other research studies in South Africa, the UK, Australia and Canada. The prevailing conclusion is that Congruent Leadership theory resonates with the experiences of colleagues, and with conference and course attendees. It complies with their experience of leading in the clinical work environment and fits with and supports their understanding of leadership from the perspective of non-titled leaders or leaders in positions without authority or managerial power.

THE LIMITATIONS OF CONGRUENT LEADERSHIP

There are limitations to Congruent Leadership theory and although it represents a new perspective on 'grassroots' leadership, the limitations should also be considered.

NEW THEORY

The research undertaken to discover and support the theory, although substantial, stands essentially alone and at this point is based on the work of the author and his research partners. While the research that supports Congruent Leadership has become significant, more research and wider exploration of the theory may still be required.

SIMILAR TO AUTHENTIC LEADERSHIP AND BREAKTHROUGH LEADERSHIP

Authentic Leadership, Breakthrough Leadership and Congruent Leadership all focus on values as the driving force for which the leader is recognised. However, similar is not the same, and it may be because Congruent Leadership has grown from a health professional focus that it rests on a firmer base to help support an understanding of leadership that is less connected to managerial and authoritarian leadership principles. Both authentic and breakthrough leadership are based on management foundations. However, as Congruent Leadership theory is grounded on and developed specifically from research undertaken in the health domain it is not just a new theory of leadership, but one based firmly on evidence with sound methodological underpinnings and health-focused research credibility. The empirical research to support both authentic and breakthrough leadership is less well developed and less well able to be linked to the actions of the leader.

NOT DRIVEN BY A SPECIFIC FOCUS ON CHANGE

Significantly, given a recent focus of leadership on vision and change, Congruent Leadership is not obvious in its focus on the promotion of leaders who are directed to 'change' practice and lead change. This does not mean that congruent leaders do not engage in innovation and change. It is just that they are not driven by this focus. An example to support this from the research undertaken that led to the theory of Congruent Leadership is from an RN who allowed a man on to a ward to sit with his ill wife outside of visiting times. The RN was reprimanded and the man ejected by the manager of the ward because the visiting time rules had been breached. The RN's actions were discussed at the subsequent ward meetings and while the manager had brought up the behaviour as an example of a staff member who had not followed ward policy, other staff recognised this RN as a congruent leader who had stood by her values in allowing the man onto the ward to comfort his wife. Her stance was along the lines of 'if I had been ill and this had been my husband, I would have wanted him with me, ward visiting hours or not.' (The man could not visit in the allotted times due to his shift work pattern.) The rest of the ward recognised the RN's values and aligned with them, putting pressure on the ward manager to consider changing their restrictive visiting time policy. It took some time and it was not the intent of the RN's actions, but after six months or so the rules regarding ward visiting time were relaxed.

It should be noted that organisational reforms across the globe are focused on better leadership for the improvement of services and products, and that leadership is being sought to support and promote change and stimulate innovation. The NHS Leadership Centre was specifically directed to promote leadership that focused very firmly on 'change' rather than 'values' centred leadership (NHS Leadership Centre, 2002) and the development of leaders who can influence people and lead change is very much a focus of much leadership concern in global organisations.

However, as Congruent Leadership is focused upon recognising the transforming power of values and meaning through actions, it can be assumed with confidence that many of the leaders' actions will result in change and innovation, motivation and inspiration, as grassroots leaders seek to (or inadvertently) influence and improve the quality of the work about them. I acknowledge, though, that organisations specifically seeking to promote leaders who drive and promote change may find Congruent Leadership too obscure for their purposes. However, I would assert that focusing on people's (or an organisation's) values and beliefs and clarifying these remains a crucial first step in any change process.

SCENARIO 5.2   CONGRUENT LEADERSHIP IN ACTION

CURRICULUM PLANNING

In 2017, I was offered an opportunity to support and lead a new Under Graduate nursing course curriculum design. I began by asking the educators involved in delivering the curriculum to start by discussing and deciding upon their key values.

This step took place before any other conversation about the course, the topics it contained or the structure and course philosophy of teaching that would underpin the way the content was delivered. For some weeks, initially through discussions and then with email collaboration and feedback, we all participated in outlining what the values we held about the focus for the course should be. It was a nursing curriculum. The values that were finally agreed upon were:

- Excellence
- Authenticity
- Care

- Compassion
- Courage
- Collaboration
- Integrity
- Diversity
- Equity

Once these were in place and everyone had had time to contribute to them, reflect upon them and agree to them, the work of building the curriculum could start. Without these values in place, the potential for significant disagreement and curriculum drift would have been strong, with individual educators pulling or pushing the curriculum in various directions. With the values in place and strongly linked to the structure and framework of the curriculum everyone involved in the following development work knew what our values were and where we stood as educators.

Building a curriculum is in itself a significant change process and this example puts values at the heart of the change process, by basing the whole process on the core values that unite (in this case) the curriculum development team.

NOT SUITABLE FOR LEADERS WITH 'CONTROL' AS AN OBJECTIVE

Leaders who are required to exercise control over others (managers) or who are not visible or engaged in the process of doing the 'work' of the people or groups (staff/employees) they lead may struggle to demonstrate a Congruent Leadership approach. Congruent leaders do not order others to adopt their values or beliefs, they display them. They stand by them and they are then evident to others, sometimes unconsciously. If leaders are in positions where they are often unable to engage in the 'work' of their colleagues, or if they are drawn into other duties or if they are required to exercise control over (manage) their colleagues or those they lead, Congruent Leadership will not be evident and may be of limited value. In the research results 'controlling' was specifically seen as a characteristic not associated with leaders who used a Congruent Leadership approach. This was commonly because a leader functioning in a position of control was seen to be placed in a position where they seemed to be a perceived 'clash of values' and as such the application of Congruent Leadership was either difficult or inappropriate.

In spite of these drawbacks, there is a significant place for Congruent Leadership in the organisational landscape. As such, I am confident that even with the above shortcomings, the results of the research and the application of Congruent Leadership theory can be used with confidence.

BASED ON RESEARCH RELATED TO THE HEALTH INDUSTRY

It could be said that a weakness of Congruent Leadership is that the theory is grounded upon research dominantly from the healthcare arena. I mention this as it may be put forward as a criticism. However, I also feel that this is a weakness only in so much as it is the sole domain of research focus, not because any leadership theory coming from the health area is itself weak. Indeed, the studies undertaken that support this theory, while all with health professionals, were undertaken in different countries, with different gender mixes, different professional groups and different methodologies and offered data gathered over many years (Bishop, 2009a, 2009b; Stanley, 2006a, 2006b, 2006c, 2006d, 2007, 2008, 2009, 2010, 2011, 2012, 2013a, , 2014, 2017; Stanley and Sherratt, 2010; Stanley and Stanley, 2017; Stanley, Cuthbertson and Latimer, 2012; Stanley, Hutton and Atkinson, 2014; : Stanley et al., 2017).

EXAMPLES OF CONGRUENT LEADERS

Joan of Arc is one of France's great national heroines. Born in 1412, she was a simple peasant girl who heard the 'voices' of saints calling her to save France from the English. With this divine inspiration she rose to become a soldier, leader, martyr and finally a saint herself. She was convinced that God had called her to free France and she showed remarkable moral courage and significant military leadership to inspire the demoralised, humiliated and discredited French army to fight on during the Hundred Years War.

Joan of Arc defied convention and the obstructions of statesmen, churchmen and generals to follow her beliefs and live out her values. Joan travelled across war-torn France to seek an audience with the Dauphin (King in waiting). She persuaded him to allow her to lead the French army to lift the Siege of Orléans. She was clad in white armour, carried a battleaxe and produced a stunning victory in only nine days.

Joan of Arc was quiet and determined, motivational and influential and had a dramatic effect on the reversal of the French army's fortunes. She was captured and given to the English during the Siege of Compiègne and was so convinced and passionate about her beliefs and values that her interrogators decided it would be useless to use torture. Nevertheless at the age of 19 she was burnt at the stake as a witch. The English were so concerned that no relic of her should remain to further inspire the French they burnt her body three times and scattered the dust from her ashes in the River Seine.

Twenty years after her death the King of France supported an inquiry into Joan of Arc's trial. The conviction was overturned and 500 years later in 1920 the Roman Catholic Church made her a Saint. Joan of Arc has remained a significant figure in French politics, and the memory of her devotion to the salvation of her country is often evoked as a political rallying cry. The story of Joan of Arc offers a contrary insight into leadership, when in an age of war and male dominance, a simple peasant girl rose to lead an army and conquer the English and their assumptions about strength and power. Joan of Arc was a Congruent Leader who stood by her values and banner to motivate, inspire and act with courage. Joan stayed true to her beliefs and values under the most trying of circumstances, but this was the very essence of her ability to motivate and command others.

In more recent times, the contribution to the campaign against domestic violence by Rose Batty can be offered as another example of Congruent Leadership. On 12 February 2014 Rose's son Luke was viciously murdered by his father. Rose had suffered ongoing domestic violence at her husband's hand and soon after her son's murder Rose began speaking out against domestic violence. Rose started actively addressing the media and government agencies about their perceptions of domestic violence and indicated that a lack of communication between services, a lack of funding and police and legal services that disempowered her ability to protect herself and her son needed to be changed. Rose established a foundation, 'The Luke Batty Foundation', to support women and children who were affected by domestic violence and Rose spoke out and campaigned for the establishment of a Royal Commission in 2015 into the challenges of family violence in Victoria, Australia.

In 2014 Rose was awarded the Pride of Australia's National Courage Medal and in 2015 she was named 'Australian of the Year'. As an advocate for the voice of women and domestic violence survivors, Rose has had a significant impact on the attitude of government agencies, on government policy and on raising the profile of a sadly all too common problem in Australian society. She has done so with dignity and clarity, courage and empathy. Rose, even while suffering the great grief of the loss of her son, found the courage and voice to address the issues of domestic violence on a platform that brought the discussion to national and international attention. In 2016 Rose was named 33rd on *Fortune* magazine's list of the World's Greatest Leaders. When faced with her son's death and after suffering years of threats and abuse, Rose's response was to put her values about what needed to be done and said into action. Rose matched her values with her actions, she stood for and spoke out in a courageous, consistent and congruent way. Rose Batty is a congruent leader.

ACTIVITY 5.1   REFLECTIVE EXERCISE

There have been a number of examples offered in the preceding chapters of congruent leaders.

Can you think of any of your own, local people, or people from your workplace, or from history who may be congruent leaders? Are you a congruent leader? What are the dominant characteristics among at least three people you have identified as a congruent leader?

CHAPTER SUMMARY

There are a number of strengths aligned with Congruent Leadership theory. These include the realisation that the theory of Congruent Leadership supports leadership at a 'grassroots' level and it helps leaders who might not have seen themselves as leaders before recognise themselves as leaders. Congruent Leadership offers a foundational leadership theory that may help leaders to build other leadership approaches and recognise the power of the link between their values and their actions. Congruent Leadership supports a greater understanding of non-positional, non-hierarchical leadership and promotes the recognition of leaders at any or all levels of an organisation across a range of interprofessional groups. Indeed, it is very clear that anyone can be a congruent leader. While there has been significant substantiation of Congruent Leadership theory, there are limitations to the theory because it is new, it appears to be similar to authentic leadership and breakthrough leadership, it is not a leadership theory driven by a specific focus on change and it is not a leadership theory for leaders with 'control' as a feature of their role.

THE
CONTEXT OF
CONGRUENT
LEADERSHIP

6

THE POWER
OF SELF

'He that would govern others, first should be the master of himself.'

Philip Massinger, English dramatist

INTRODUCTION

Knowing our values begins with knowing ourselves. When Shakespeare wrote the following words in *Hamlet* (Act I, Scene 3, line 78) in 1601, 'This above all: to thine own self be true, And it must follow, as the night the day, Thou canst not then be false to any man.' Shakespeare may really have been speaking of the power of our true self as an authentic tool for the deliverance of congruence. What is important to us, what our aspirations are, how we relate to or interact with others and mostly how well we know who we are and what matters as we pass through life matter as we lead. This chapter is about strategies that may be useful in terms of helping us understand who we are, what we value and how this impacts on our relationships with others. Fundamentally this chapter explores the relationship of 'self' in establishing effective Congruent Leadership. To achieve this, this chapter will explore a number of steps that support an understanding of Congruent Leadership and how the 'self' is pivotal to how congruent leaders act. The chapter concludes by exploring further examples of congruent leaders who display their values and beliefs and who lead by matching the values and beliefs, with their actions.

WHO ARE YOU?

In Mary Gentile's (2010) excellent book, *Giving Voice to Values*, she starts by suggesting that in many Eastern philosophies and in martial arts practice, strength comes from harnessing our momentum and energy and moving with it rather than against it, thus using the force of momentum to supplement our own energy. This is similar to understanding how Congruent Leadership can build leadership potential, where acting in concert with our values creates greater power and energy than voice or actions alone. So, how do we know ourselves?

PERSONALITY

We could start by understanding our individual personality. Personality is commonly described as the way a person responds to situations, or a person's preferred way of behaving in particular situations. Hall and Lindzey (1957) describe our personality as a fairly consistent characteristic pattern of thoughts, feelings and behaviours that make a person unique. Warren and Carmichael (1930, p. 333) also suggest that 'personality is the entire mental organisation of a human being at any stage of his [*sic*] development. It embraces every phase of human character: intellect, temperament, skill, morality, and every attitude that has been built up in the course of one's life.'

So significant has become an understanding of our personality and its influence on who we are and why we do what we do that there is substantial research into personality types. In addition, a number of tools or indicators have been designed to help us, as well as psychologists and employers (in some cases), to learn more about who we are. These generally fall into the field of psychometric testing and you may have been subjected to some or heard of some of the more common tools for exploring personality types. The Myers-Briggs Type Indicator (MBTI) is possibly the most well known. This tool explains our work style and our preference for responses at work and in interpersonal situations, and supports an understanding of our preferred communication strategies, leadership styles and decision-making processes. Other tools, such as the California Psychological Inventory (CPI) and the Fundamental Interpersonal Relations Orientation-Behaviour (FIROB), are possibly less well known but remain well used, and of course there are yet others (they can all be located with a simple web search). All of these tools offer usually well tested and tried approaches with simple questionnaires that allow generally self-selecting options, leading to insights into various aspects of our preferred personality type.

I am most familiar with Myers-Briggs and it is, if nothing else, interesting in the scope and depth of the analysis offered. The criticism of this tool (and all the others) is that it is reductionist in its application, so that with Myers-Briggs, everyone is classified into 16 one-off, personality types. That simply may not capture the rich and diverse tapestry of human personalities. However, if you are searching for help in answering the 'Who am I?' question, these tools and others offer a useful place to start. Few of the tools have been rigorously tested in a standardised way, and a study by Janowsky, et al. in 2002 found that as many as 75 per cent of people who took the Myers-Briggs Type Indicator assessment were assigned different personality types on subsequent attempts.

Covey (1989) suggests that there are seven habits of highly effective leaders, although he also suggests that the greatest asset we have in terms of leadership is ourself. Covey (1989) recommends the establishment of a balance between the physical, emotional, social and mental sides of our nature. To do so he recommends paying attention to each dimension of our self. This too requires a degree of insight into who we are. Chade-Meng (2013) also suggests that searching inside ourselves is a vital step in terms of recognising ourselves and realising our full potential.

So, are there other approaches to understanding who we are and why we do what we do? There are debates about nature and nurture and the influence these have on our personality types. There are discussions about the influence of gender, culture, education and life events that impact upon us as we grow. The reality is we are all different, and different again in a range of contexts – who we are in the comfort of our own home may be different from who we are on the sports field or at work or in a professional role, but there are things that unite us. Gentile (2010, p. 1) suggests we need to take an enabling stance in which, rather than trying to pull or push ourselves into a values-based set of actions, we should be trying to 'grease the skids that might carry us there'. This means we should identify the times when we already know how to act in accord with our highest moral values and the reasons we feel the way we do at these times. Then we need to focus on building our confidence and competence or develop strong internal scripts that enable us to act effortlessly and with the least personal disquiet. In this way we work with rather than against our personal momentum, falling back on a set of practised and well-worn actions and negating the rationalisations and pre-emptive arguments that filter into our values-based decisions and actions. Gentile (2010 p. 2) suggests that this approach 'creates a safe and enabling space' to test and create our values and begin to explore who we are.

Or you could simply ask your family, your friends, your workmates and indeed any one you trust to give you a fair and honest answer. We generally spend time with and invest our interest in people whose values and beliefs we align with. So, most of us are on pretty safe ground to start with. It almost goes without saying that the people we like, the people we spend time around, the people we mix with at work and the people we play sport with or mix with socially are the best reflection of who we are. Facebook and other social media platforms are fun and interesting but they seem less helpful in this context. People who do not know you, who may know only one small aspect of who you are or what you do, will not be able to offer a great deal of insight into the person you are or the values you hold. Far too many people take on board the positive and (more importantly) the negative feedback they get from random strangers who may troll them or bully them, often expressing their own ignorance and prejudice in the process. This is important because, as Gentile (2010) indicates, the better we know ourselves, the more we can prepare to play to our strengths and, when necessary, protect ourselves from any weaknesses we may have.

ACTIVITY 6.1   REFLECTIVE EXERCISE

Ask your friends, family or workmates to give you a frank evaluation of what they think motivates or drives you.

Do you agree? Does their view match your own idea or perception of yourself? Why do you think they may be different?

There is power in knowing who we are, in identifying what it is about each of us that enables us to respond to various situations one way or another. There is power in recognising that our values unite us and can be a force for increasing our momentum when seeking to make ethical decisions or move away from situations we recognise as contrary to our values or beliefs. There are other approaches to exploring who we are and why a values-based leadership approach such as Congruent Leadership may be useful. Some of these are explored further in the pages below.

FINDING YOUR TRUE VOICE

Kouzes and Posner (2010) suggest that the first step on any leadership journey is to find your own true voice. What they are suggesting is that you have to choose your own values. The second step they suggest is to listen, observe and understand other people's values. Gentile (2010) takes this further by suggesting that values-based leadership is about learning to be more of who we really are rather than learning to become other than who we are. Gentile (2010, p. xv) adds that leading ethically is not just about 'deciding what the right thing to do is', but it is about knowing 'how to get it done'. This perspective lines up well with the concept of Congruent Leadership and supports my contention that to understand values-based leadership (Congruent Leadership) we need to start by understanding ourselves.

Personal values drive commitment. You can only commit to an organisation, political action, personal ambition, professional progression or indeed anything if there is a fit between what you are doing and what you value and believe. To lead effectively means being aware of what you believe, what your values are and where you stand. Clearly, belief alone is not enough. There must also be evidence, grown from research in the application of your work or profession. There must also be a commitment to breach the gap between what is known and what might be known, and there also needs to be a desire to be open and honest. Congruent leaders also need to act with dignity, respect and professionalism in communicating or proposing a change, innovation or a new way to look at the world. They need to be resilient, courageous, calm and passionate, and foster a robust sense of humour. Finally, a Congruent Leader also needs to be knowledgeable, visible and act as a positive role model for the change or innovation being suggested or discussed. Once these features are established or clear, progress may be made towards their development. It is possible to change a work practice, a personal trait, the way we respond to people, the way we look at problems, the way we interact with others, how we communicate, how we react to change ... how we see or are 'present' in the world.

WIDEN YOUR VIEW

This step involves recognising that change is possible just by knowing where you stand. It links with an understanding of empowerment. Empowerment can be seen one way, as a process by which we facilitate the participation of others in decision-making or taking action. Empowerment expressed this way can be seen as an ability to exert influence through the possession of knowledge or skills that are useful to others. I am not a fan of this perspective. It implies that one person can empower another. I do not believe this to be the case. I believe others can motivate us, teach us, stimulate us, coerce us, bribe us, bully us, force us or trick and manipulate us into doing what they want. However, real empowerment rests within us all and can only really be activated by the individual who chooses to be empowered.

I suggest that the application of 50,000 volts may stimulate a person to respond or perform or confess, but it will not empower them. Empowerment, according to Rogers (1979), comes from personal growth and this leads to personal power and so to empowerment. In the end people can choose to be or not to be empowered. As mentioned in Chapter 3, Mandela faced copious obstacles in his path to the leadership of South Africa. His autobiography is called *A Long Walk to Freedom*. This was because it was him taking action that led to freedom. It was not a 'long road', a 'long journey' or a 'long drive' to freedom, but a walk. It was him, taking his own steps. It was not the sort of 'empowerment' that was given, imposed, transferred, taught or injected. I cannot empower you to understand Congruent Leadership. To do this you need to act, to read the book, to reflect, to do something that I cannot make you do, although I may suggest actions and interventions. As with any attempt to give up an addiction the power to do so needs to come from within the person and it places the power to act or to make a choice squarely with the individual (I call it 'me-powerment').

Not convinced? Read about or think about people you might know who could be congruent leaders or the people discussed in the various chapters of this book. Not one of them waited at home for empowerment to be delivered by Amazon. They found their values and acted on them themselves, with a power that came from within. Congruent leaders are empowered.

BECOME MORE EMOTIONALLY INTELLIGENT

Emotional intelligence is not a new concept. Although not the first to describe what emotional intelligence is, Goleman (1998) was certainly one of the most prominent writers on this topic. However, Salovey and Mayer (1990) describe emotional intelligence as our ability to monitor our own and others' feelings and emotions, to discriminate among them and to use this information to guide our actions and thinking. Goleman (1998) supports this, stating that emotional intelligence is our capacity for recognising our own feelings and those of others, it is our ability to motivate ourselves and effectively deal with our own and others' emotions. Goleman (1998) makes it clear that emotions are an essential part of who we are and that our ability to express our emotions (or not) at the right time and in the right way or place is a concern for most people. Emotional intelligence is our capacity to determine when to address our and others' emotions and when to 'park' them (Brockbank and McGill, 2007).

Many people react to a range of life events with their emotions, claiming they were unable to control them. Feelings of betrayal, regret, anger, jealousy, fear, loss, hurt or feeling let down, or indeed positive emotions such as, happiness, joy and elation, are common emotions that may be claimed were too raw to be contained. However, emotional intelligence is expressed as the person's ability to exercise control over these emotions, not so they are suppressed or ignored, but so that the response is measured by a conscious acknowledgement of the feelings we may be experiencing.

Goleman (2005) suggested there are five building blocks for emotional intelligence. These are:

1. *Self-awareness* – the ability to understand and monitor our own emotions and to recognise the influence they have on our performance at work and impact on our relationships.
2. *Self-management (or self-regulation)* – our ability to exercise self-control and be conscious of our emotions.
3. *Social awareness (expressed as empathy)* – our ability to sense the emotions of others, to understand their perspective and be sensitive to their feelings and reactions.
4. *Social skills* – these are a set of skills related to communication and confidence that help facilitate listening and relationship-building skills. Social skills help us build bonds and cooperate or work with others productively.
5. *Motivation* – this is the will to go beyond any superficial connections and to build successful and meaningful personal and professional relationships. It expresses a willingness to commit to more than yourself.

Emotional intelligence is about exercising self-control, applying zeal and persistence in motivating oneself, sometimes in the face of frustrations. Emotional intelligence is connected to delayed gratification, monitoring and regulating one's mood and keeping distress away from our ability to think. For congruent leaders monitoring and controlling their emotions is essential as they are meant to serve us and not control us. As such, emotional intelligence helps congruent leaders recognise that emotions can help our well-being, but only if they are employed appropriately. Instead of trying to avoid emotions especially at work, congruent leaders have an important role in providing support and guidance that harness the energy of emotional interactions positively (Rajah et al., 2011; Taylor et al., 2015). Goleman et al. (2013) suggest that when it comes to shaping our decisions and actions, feelings count every bit as much as our thoughts, if not more so as congruent leaders are recognised by their actions.

Self-awareness is the key to the development of emotional intelligence as it facilitates our recognition of our feelings and moods as well as the thoughts about our mood or what drives them. Being attuned to our emotions also helps us recognise the emotions of others. This leads to the next key in the development of emotional intelligence: the development of empathy and our ability to recognise the often subtle social signals that help us understand another's needs or wants. Once developed, emotional intelligence can help congruent leaders manage relationships well which leads to more effective interpersonal and professional or workplace relationships. It also leads to more effective leadership and being better able to manage conflict successfully (Antonakis et al., 2009; Taylor et al., 2015).

The benefits of developing and employing an emotionally intelligent leadership approach is that congruent leaders will know their feelings and use them to make key decisions they can live with. They will be better informed about their level of self-awareness, they will know what triggers or 'pushes' their buttons. They will not be overwhelmed by worry or anger and they will persist in pursuing their leadership, professional, workplace and personal goals despite occasional setbacks (Por et al., 2011). They will be able to handle feelings and relationships with skill and maturity (Taylor et al., 2015) and be able to moderate the impact of stressful situations on their mental health (Benson et al., 2010). Congruent leaders are able to use communication strategies effectively to be able to influence the quality of the work they do and the relationships they build. As such, they will be able to manage clear communication in a crisis which may be central to clarifying and resolving disputes. Remaining calm and in control may have immediate effects and, finally, improving their communication and conflict management styles will help build rapport and mean that congruent leaders are better able to get the job done (Taylor et al., 2015).

ISLANDS

No person is an island … emotional intelligence is not just about being nice to ourselves and others, it is about making choices about how we feel, identifying emotions in others and providing the support needed to bolster and build relationships and connections. This can have a dramatic impact on the success of our work and personal relationships and ultimately on our ability to advance in our career or grow as people (Taylor et al., 2015). The principles of interprofessional working support this perspective. Client or patient safety and effective communication in the health service are based upon a premise that different professional disciplines will be able to work in teams with each other and not in isolation. It is often said that a great résumé will get you the interview and that intelligence will get you the job, but it is effective emotional intelligence that will keep you in the job and connected to the people around you. It is also the congruent leader who understands and applies emotional intelligence that will find followers who are loyal and forgiving and aligned to the leader's values. The good news is that emotional intelligence can be learnt and developed over time (Goleman, 2005).

A final note on the link between congruent leaders and emotional intelligence is the concept that a leader's values and beliefs are deemed to be more visible when they are demonstrated in practice. Leaders who are congruent in their actions facilitate constructive emotional responses that are conducive and effective in a variety of interactions and situations. Emotionally competent leaders who are able to regulate their emotions confidently and are able to motivate others by sharing collective values and beliefs that impact positively in all environments are more effective (Bulmer Smith et al., 2009; Heckeman et al., 2015). Goleman et al. (2013) suggest that the emotional task of a leader is 'primal' because it is both original and the most important act of leadership. Congruent leaders lead through their actions and are therefore capable of inspiring and motivating others towards achieving desirable outcomes and developing innovative practices, if linked and consistent with their well-managed emotions.

EMPATHY

To some extent this was covered as an attribute of emotional intelligence. However, I have singled it out as I feel it has a special place in the development and application of Congruent Leadership, specifically for health professionals. The power of empathy is that it facilitates connections, whereas sympathy may drive disconnection. Wiseman (1996) suggests that there are four qualities or attributes of empathy. The first is perspective taking or our ability to look at an issue, problem or situation from another's perspective. The second is to refrain from judgement, recognising the emotions of others and then being able to communicate our understanding of the emotion. These offer strong links to emotional intelligence and the principles of interprofessional working, but there is something more primal about our ability to express empathy. At its core, empathy is our ability to feel 'with' people. This sits comfortably with congruent leaders who are present, visible and able to 'be' with others.

I really like the word 'midwife'. I used to be one (indeed I am still registered to practise as a midwife). The reason I like the word is because it describes the word's meaning. Midwife means 'with women'. It doesn't mean baby deliverer, it doesn't mean nurse and it doesn't mean child carer. Being 'with women' is what midwives do. Midwives are there at the woman's side, with women throughout the pregnancy, labour, birth and post-partum period. Midwives are with the new-born too, but primarily midwives are with the woman and in more modern times with the husband, father and family too. In a powerful way the word 'midwife' is an expression of empathy, one of being in a role that is visible and present, connected.

CONNECTION

Empathy is a choice and it is a risky one to take because it means having to connect to something within ourselves that allows us to really reach out to or connect with or take another's perspective, non-judgementally. The power of empathy is in the choice we make to establish a connection. Congruent leaders make this choice each time they stand resolutely by their values and each time they put into practice the actions that support or signal their values. Not being able to connect to others will weaken our capacity to lead and, in a very real way, break or fail to support the bonds with followers. Many congruent leaders make these connections subconsciously. As they are approachable, courageous and passionate, persistent, determined, energetic and positive they are open to expressions of empathy and others (followers) are attracted to them. Being closed to our own emotions, being closed to the power we have within ourselves and our ability to form powerful connections with others, will weaken the congruent leader's ability to lead clearly, resolutely and with confidence.

RESILIENCE

Not everyone will hold or believe in the values you have. Many will try and bring you down, undermine your stance or steal your voice. Many will simply hold to a different set of values. Dillard (1993, p. 126) refers to resilience as 'hardiness' and describes it as the leader's ability to 'withstand or adapt to change and stress'. Resilience is built upon commitment and fed by endurance and persistence. Resilient leaders are able to weather the slings and arrows of change and to cope with environmental or organisational change, change in managers and a change in supervision because they ground the strength of their resilience in their values. In support of this view, Dillard (1993, p. 127) suggests that the 'characteristics basic to an effective and hardy leader include coherence and consistency in beliefs and values'.

Being able to hold a stance or position and resiliently stand by our values requires courage and perseverance. It does not mean that compromise is off the table, but does imply that leaders need to be clear about what their values are, what they should resolutely stand for and what can be negotiated. Congruent leaders need to use emotional intelligence and ethical principles to determine which values they should hold like a sword and which they should drop like a stone. Determining which is which is one of the great challenges we each face and beyond the scope of this book to explore, although the ones we hold on to need to be held with determination and strength.

In many workplaces bullying and sociopathic behaviour may be a manifestation of values that have become detached from ethical principles and the sound application of emotional intelligence. In some workplaces some people are not just unkind to others, they actively seek to undermine, belittle or destroy others' harmony, comfort or contribution. These sorts of behaviours require resilience of a remarkable degree and in some cases the wisest choice is to work somewhere else, especially if your resilience is being pushed beyond tolerable levels. This is not failure and is usually the result of incompatible values or intolerable behaviours. Congruent leaders may want to persist and demonstrate their commitment to their values, they may want to put on a show of their resilience and in normal circumstances this is appropriate.

One example is the treatment of Desmond Doss, an American infantry man who was bullied, beaten and ridiculed by his peers and officers in the hope he would leave the army voluntarily. This was because Doss was a 'conscientious objector' and while he wanted to serve as a medic, his religious beliefs and personal values meant that he did not want to carry a gun or shoot people. He survived an attempt to have him discharged from the Army and persevered through the mistreatment, aggression and ridicule of his 'comrades'. Eventually he was allowed to serve as a medic and he travelled with his company to the Pacific Ocean theatre in the Second World War where he took part in the Okinawa campaign. There he served in the battle for Hacksaw Ridge on the Maeda Escarpment. His company suffered significant losses, but Doss was involved in retrieving wounded and injured soldiers (on both sides) often without help. Over the course of an evening and night, still under enemy fire and without rest, Doss rescued 75 men and was subsequently nominated for and received the Medal of Honor, the highest military decoration of the USA armed forces.

Described by a *Telegraph* review as a 'man askew' (Hawkes, 2017), Doss proved to be physically and emotionally resilient. He was courageous and determined, not just in the battle, but in the face of his mistreatment from many men that he was later to save. Doss was a congruent leader, because when given an opportunity to put his values into action he did so courageously and with significant conviction.

In the workplace we are often called upon to be almost as resilient, dealing with corporate policies and behaviours that fail to render fair or compassionate treatment to customers, clients, service users, employees, staff or subcontractors. I have been told the workplace is not meant to be fair or compassionate. I disagree. Values that help build connections, facilitate integrity, honesty, trust, respect and compassion have to be better places to work, happier places to be innovative, safer places to experiment and places more appropriate for feeling secure. Congruent leaders, who role model resilience and practise beliefs and behaviours that foster values that support better places to work, should be the gold standard in our industry, institutions and organisations.

EXAMPLES OF CONGRUENT LEADERS

The life and deeds of Mother Teresa (known in the Catholic Church as Saint Teresa of Calcutta) was an Albanian-Indian Roman Catholic nun and missionary who can be cited as another example of a congruent leader. She was resolute and empathetic, and she found her voice and stood by her values to courageously change the health and life outcomes for many people because she applied her values and beliefs to her actions. When Agnes Gonxha Bojaxhiu (later known as 'Mother Teresa') set off for Darjeeling in 1929 to join the Sisters of Loreto she was originally assigned the role of teacher at St Mary's High School, where she taught for 15 years. However, in 1946 she received what she described as 'a call from God' to give up her teaching role and 'follow Christ into the slums to serve him among the poorest of the poor'. She undertook some medical training and after many obstacles were overcome, she set up the Missionaries of Charity order, who took a fourth vow, to give free help to the poorest people (the original three vows are poverty, chastity and obedience).

Her mission, in her words, was to 'care for the hungry, the naked, the homeless, the crippled, the blind, the lepers, all those who feel unwanted, unloved, uncared for throughout society, people that have become a burden to society and are shunned by everyone'. The first of the Order's centres opened in Calcutta and from there others gradually spread across India. Mother Teresa was to be honoured with some of the world's greatest awards, but it remained her beliefs and values that centred her life. 'Love', she said, 'begins at home and it is not how much we do, but how much love we put in the action(s) that we do.' Mother Teresa is another example of a congruent leader. It could be argued that she is the very definition of a congruent leader, because her life was lived as a very testament to her values and beliefs.

Mother Teresa's approach to leadership may not even have been seen as leadership yet she inspired millions of people. She established a new religious Order and with empathy, courage and personal empowerment set up and supported her mission, often with limited help and financial support. It is this type of leadership that is fundamentally based on a link between the leader's values and beliefs and their actions. Ultimately leading is about what we do. Congruent Leadership may not define a person's life the way it did Mother Teresa's, but the principles of Congruent Leadership do offer an explanation of how and why leaders are able to do what they do and are followed in the way they are. However, Congruent Leadership is not the same as religious devotion.

Another example of a congruent leader, this time from a medical perspective, is the life of Ernest Edward (Weary) Dunlop (Ebury, 1994; Edwards, 2011). He began his career as a pharmacist but gained a scholarship to study medicine at the University of Melbourne in 1927. He graduated with a Bachelor of Medicine and Bachelor of Surgery in 1934. He was also an excellent sportsman and represented his country at rugby in 1932 and his university at boxing. At the outbreak of the Second World War he joined the Australian Army Medical Corps with the rank of captain.

In 1942 he was sent to Indonesia to treat Australian troops, but was captured by the Japanese and was sent with the troops to Thailand, where the prisoners were forced to begin work on the Burma–Thailand railway (soon to be known as 'the railway of death'). Dunlop became the commanding and medical officer at the prisoner of war (POW) camps in Java, Changi (in Singapore) and Thailand. As he did so he inspired prisoners with his compassion, dedication to duty, medical skills and knowledge. He is credited with numerous selfless and heroic acts, often in defiance of the Japanese captors that went well beyond the responsibilities of his role as an officer.

The living conditions in the camps were atrocious, with rampant tropical disease, inadequate food, poor shelter and brutality from the work schedule and their captors. Medical supplies were scarce, but Weary stretched them where he could or improvised from other materials when possible. One of 'Weary's thousand' troops, Don Stuart, wrote of him: 'When despair and death reached us, Weary Dunlop stood fast ... he was a lighthouse of sanity in a universe of madness and suffering.'

However, it wasn't his vision or creativity or authority that attracted the troops to follow and respect him. It was his capacity to live (even in the trying and deadly conditions of the POW camps) in accord with his personal values and beliefs, securing the trust of the troops and letting them know that he was with them and would not abandon them. Caring for the ill and wounded in the face of significant challenges and great personal risk, he was a role model, acting with humanity and dignity. Visible, courageous, determined, knowledgeable and competent – lesser men might have resorted to authority and power, collaboration for resources and greed or the serving of their own self-interests. Weary Dunlop, however, largely maintained morale and succeeded in maintaining a reasonable survival rate that compared well against other nations' prisoner populations in the Asian region.

As with Mother Teresa, Weary Dunlop was to receive numerous awards and commendations in the years after the war and he worked hard to build better relations between Asian nations and Australia. He also worked tirelessly for better support for war veterans and helped establish the Sir Edward Dunlop Medical Research Foundation. Weary Dunlop is another example of a congruent leader, matching his values and beliefs with his actions.

CHAPTER SUMMARY

This chapter has offered information about the significance of understanding who we are and how this may impact upon or is impacted upon our values and beliefs. It is suggested that knowing who we are and what our values are is fundamental to being an effective congruent leader. Understanding what makes us who we are, our personality and our strengths and weaknesses may help each of us to lead or follow more effectively. There are established tools to help explore personality types; however, we can also seek insight from our friends and families and people who know us well or that we trust. To develop as a congruent leader, it is proposed that it is important to find our true voice or understand the values we stand by. We should widen our view and seek to realise that empowerment is already within us all, we should foster our emotional intelligence and seek to connect with people empathetically. In addition, congruent leaders need to practise and show resilience and courage, and to stand by their values in the face of often stern opposition or ridicule.

If we are to be true 'to thine own self', we need to start by being open to gaining insight into who we are and why knowing this is connected to the significance of our values. Only then will we have the capacity to stand firmly on the foundations of our values and hold strongly to the standard of our principles for others to see.

7

ORGANISATIONAL CULTURE AND CONGRUENT LEADERSHIP

'Values aren't buses ... they're not supposed to get you anywhere. They're supposed to define who you are.'

Jennifer Crusie, author

INTRODUCTION

This chapter addresses the relationship between organisational culture, leadership and the vital role of Congruent Leadership in helping leaders shape or influence an organisation's culture. In the introduction to a health-related publication, *Culture of Care Barometer* by Rafferty et al. (2015, p. 6), it is made clear 'that quality and culture are not uniform within let alone across organisations.' As a result, the lack of consistency in 'culture(s) impedes the spread of good practice across organisations' (Rafferty et al., 2015 p.6). They add that, in the main, organisational, 'failures are not usually brought to light by the systems ... such as incidence reporting, mortality and morbidity reviews, inspections, accreditations clinical profiling and risk and claim management' (Rafferty et al., 2015, p. 6). This is because these metrics fail to capture the reality for most patients, clients and health professional staff. Instead, it is only by understanding and influencing the 'culture of care' that genuine change and improvements can be made, with culture being seen as everybody's business and central to the way things are done within each organisation. These comments relate to the health industry; however, they can be applied equally to any business or organisation.

As congruent leaders are firmly focused on putting into practice their values, and as values are an open expression of culture, there is a direct link between the activity of congruent leaders and their influence and impact on an organisation's culture (or indeed any area where a culture is evident). The chapter concludes by exploring further examples of congruent leaders and describing the implications for recognising leaders who lead by matching their values and beliefs with their actions.

WHAT IS ORGANISATIONAL CULTURE?

Organisational culture is not an easy concept to pin down and has been described as a vague and hard to grasp concept at best, with many organisations unsure of what it is and how to change or guide it (Neuhauser, 2005). However, it signifi-cantly influences all aspects of any organisation. Schein (2014) defines culture as:

> A pattern of shared basic assumptions that the group learned as it solved its problems of external adaption and internal integration, that has worked well enough to be considered valid and, therefore, to be taught to new members as the correct way to perceive, think, and feel in relation to those problems. (Schein, 2014, p. 17)

Schein (2014, p. 17) referred to his definition as 'an empirically based abstraction' and a search of current literature suggests a number of other definitions and descriptions of organisational culture. One of the simplest and most common expressions of organisational culture is simply, 'How things are done around here' (Fowke, 1999, p. 1). Another understanding of organisational culture is that it is 'The pattern of beliefs, values and learned ways of coping with experience that have developed during the course of an organisation's history, and which tend to be manifest in its material arrangements and in the behaviours of its members' (Brown, 1995, cited in S. Sun, 2008, p. 137). Helmreich and Merritt (2005) describe the organisational culture as the 'values, beliefs, rituals, symbols and behaviours that we share with others and that help define us as a group, especially in relation to other groups' (Helmreich and Merritt, 2005, p. 1).

Hall (2005) aids our understanding of organisational culture by suggesting that every organisation, regardless of its size, age or industry, has a culture. Hall (2005) adds that leading organisations are separated from each other by their ability to shape or direct the culture to bolster their business or support the organisation to better achieve their goals and engage the 'hearts and minds' of their employees, or create an environment where people are inspired to achieve extraordinary results (Hall, 2005, p. 1). In summary, it can be said that an organisation, an institution and a business culture are systems of shared values held by members of the organisation. These are commonly known, shared, communicated and held to be the features that distinguish organisations, institutions or businesses from one another.

Davies et al. (2000) support this by suggesting that there are two ways to conceptualise organisational culture. Firstly, organisational culture can be seen as something that an organisation 'is'. Culture, seen this way, indicates that the social interaction of people within the culture make the organisation and become the organisation. The second view of organisational culture is that an organisation 'has' a culture and that it is part of but separate from the organisation, in effect an attribute (Davies et al., 2000; Scott et al., 2003).

Seen this second way, it is possible to see organisational culture as something that can be modified, created or even managed (Davies et al., 2000). Hofstede and Bond (1984, p. 170) offer a different view and define organisational culture as a collective programming of the mind which differentiates the members of one human group from another.

Hofstede and Bond (1984) developed a model called 'culture dimensions' to describe the impact of a society's culture on the values of its population. The culture dimensions were developed as a consequence of applying a factor analysis to investigate the results of a worldwide survey by IBM (a leading computer company at the time) conducted between 1978 and 1983. According to this view, people are predominantly affected by their own society, which can also impact upon their attitudes towards work and their understanding of their work. Hofstede and Bond's (1984) view places culture in a place of being fundamental to an organisation and suggests that it has a powerful influence on employee (human) behaviour. As such, understanding or shaping organisational culture occupies a powerful place in the development of a highly successful organisation.

Wei et al. (2009) describe four stages in which cultures may develop or be related to the workplace:

- *Stage 1*. The values, beliefs, aspirations and vision of the organisation. These are used as an inspiration or driver to translate the manager's or leader's assumptions into values and then to symbols.
- *Stage 2*. This is where values are embedded into the system, practice and policies of the organisation.
- *Stage 3*. When maturation occurs as a result of negotiations with the drivers. Maturation is reached when the organisation becomes stable and the subculture(s) of the organisation are defined. Ultimately, the meaning of values are changed based on the outcome of the negotiations and the new artefacts.
- *Stage 4*. Finally, transformation occurs. This is the result of the restoration of the basic assumptions to the new unified area of growth. While culture is invisible and operates outside the awareness of people, leaders should understand it at the organisational level to avoid possible conflicts that can negatively affect work practices.

The analogy of an iceberg is often used to represent the 'seen' and 'unseen' elements within an organisational culture. The 'seen' elements are described as the surface manifestations of the culture (rites and rituals) which are commonly thought to be more readily manipulated and open to change. The 'unseen' elements represent the deeper beliefs, feelings and values that are often below the surface, unseen and far more difficult to recognise or change. It is these deeper elements that are described as a reflection of the values of an organisation and these point to the organisation's approach to key issues such as safety, quality, productivity, communication and attitudes to the employees and people who interact with or use the service or products.

However, there is far more to organisational culture than the definitions let on. An organisation's culture (as with any culture) is deeply embedded and grown from shared emotional experiences that are often unconscious and made up of shared basic assumptions and beliefs which guide how people relate to each other. From this initial outline it can be seen that there are clear links between the application of Congruent Leadership and shaping and developing an organisation's culture.

Understanding culture also helps members of the culture recognise their identity or membership within the culture. Seeing leadership from one perspective (that it is tied to a management function) means that people who might be legitimate leaders or be potential leaders are not recognised as such, because the cultural norms fail to recognise leadership in a wider set of terms. This links back to an earlier discussion in Chapter 5 about being able to name leaders who might not fit a traditional leadership model of being authoritarian, in a management position, powerful or titled.

TYPES OF ORGANISATIONAL CULTURE

Cameron and Quinn (2011) developed a Competing Values Framework with four major cultural types: market culture, hierarchy culture, clan culture and adhocracy culture (see Figure 7.1). These four culture types are based on four criteria: stability and control; flexibility and discretion; internal focus and integration; and external focus and differentiation, with each type characterised by a set of principles.

- *The market culture* has a strong external focus and a results-based organisation. Employees within this culture are aggressively competitive and focused on goals. Its main purpose is to increase productivity, profits, success, reputation and customer satisfaction (e.g. in a private cosmetic procedure clinic).
- *The hierarchy culture* has strong internal focus and is known for its structured work environment. Employees work under reliable internal procedures and control mechanisms. Leaders are the main coordinators and organisers and improvement strategies are usually based on error detection (e.g. a large metropolitan hospital).
- *The clan culture* is similar to being in an extended family and is characterised by its internal focus and the flexibility of the values. The clan culture encourages cooperation between people, supports organised teamwork, and is concerned with the safety of people and open communication. It also emphasises people development and bonds employees by morals. The leader's role is to facilitate, mentor and build teams (e.g. a small rural or remote health centre).

- *The adhocracy culture* has an external focus and flexibility in values and is described as a dynamic, continuous improvement and creative working place. Employees take risks and leaders are innovators and risk takers. This culture responds rapidly to changes in the outside environment. Within the organisation, experiments and innovation are the bonding materials (e.g. a private clinic or GP service).

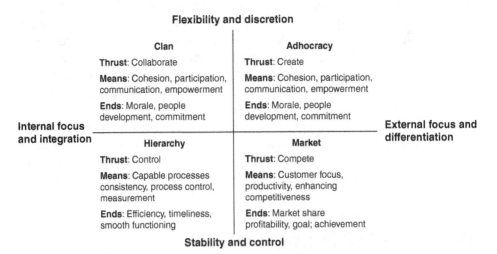

Flexibility and discretion

	Clan	Adhocracy
	Thrust: Collaborate	**Thrust**: Create
	Means: Cohesion, participation, communication, empowerment	**Means**: Cohesion, participation, communication, empowerment
	Ends: Morale, people development, commitment	**Ends**: Morale, people development, commitment

Internal focus and integration ——————————————————— **External focus and differentiation**

	Hierarchy	Market
	Thrust: Control	**Thrust**: Compete
	Means: Capable processes consistency, process control, measurement	**Means**: Customer focus, productivity, enhancing competitiveness
	Ends: Efficiency, timeliness, smooth functioning	**Ends**: Market share profitability, goal; achievement

Stability and control

Figure 7.1   Competing values framework

Source: Cameron and Quinn (2011, p. 32). Reproduced with permission of John Wiley & Sons.

ORGANISATIONAL CULTURE LEVELS

In 1980, Schein examined organisational culture and developed a model to describe the culture and make it more visible within an organisation. He described organisational culture as having three levels: (1) artefacts and symbols; (2) espoused values and beliefs; and (3) basic underlying assumptions (see Figure 7.2). These levels describe the extent to which organisational culture could be perceived and are sometimes referred to as the 'onion model'. As with the iceberg model, artefacts and symbols refer to the visible elements of the organisation (to the employees and external users). Artefacts could include the organisation's logo, uniform and structure. Although this level may be easy to identify and describe, it may be difficult to decipher. The second level of an organisation's culture was described by Schein (2014) as the espoused beliefs and values. These are characterised by standards, values and rules of conduct championed by leaders at all levels. Problems or issues can arise when the views and ideas of managers or leaders are in conflict with the basic assumptions of the organisation. The final level of an organisation's culture relates to the basic underlying assumptions. These may be deeply embedded and long established as organisational traditions within the culture of an organisation and they are commonly the original source of the organisation's values. It is at this level that people's behaviour is shaped within the organisations.

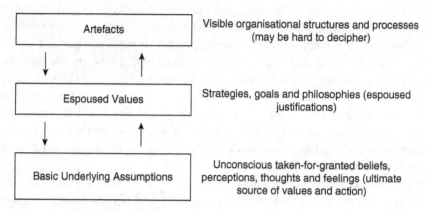

Figure 7.2   Organisational culture levels

Culture also offers a source of stability within an organisation, helping employees, staff, customers, students, teachers, patients and clients recognise where their place is in the complex structures and systems of a large organisation. Culture is based on often unquestioned assumptions about values and beliefs, with each member of the organisation's culture commonly fitting in because they don't even realise that they are working towards shared basic assumptions and core common beliefs. This may go some way to explaining why some congruent leaders don't recognise that it is their shared values and beliefs that mark them out as leaders. Cultures are built from pivotal events (ceremonies, stories, myths and key events) that form the bedrock of shared beliefs and values. As such, it is values and beliefs that are used to build an organisation's culture and again this is why an appreciation of Congruent Leadership is so vital.

An organisational culture can be built or made by design (or default), implying that if a culture is not designed, consciously constructed or structured with intent it will grow and become embedded of its own accord through the power and influence of members of the organisation or subcultures within the larger organisation. Cultures, like those in a science lab dish, will grow of their own accord, but they can also be nurtured and directed to grow in specific ways depending on the nutrients we offer.

There is a Native American Cherokee story about a child who asks a wise chief about what drives us. He explains that within us all there are two wolves, each competing for our soul. It is a terrible and ongoing fight. The chief explains: one is evil – this wolf is regret, anger, greed, sorrow, envy, arrogance, self-pity, fear, resentment, inferiority, guilt, lies, false pride, superiority and ego; the other wolf is good – generosity, truth, compassion, joy, peace, love, hope, serenity, humility, kindness, benevolence, empathy and faith. This fight is going on inside us all, he explains. The child thinks for a moment and asks, 'Which wolf will win?' The wise Cherokee chief simply replies, 'The one you feed.'

An organisation's culture grows and thrives (or not) in the same way. Culture is a social energy built over time and it is something that can also change over time. Indeed, organisational cultures are always changing, as new staff, new employees, new managers, new circumstances and new politics or policies come to play on the goals, values, direction and actions of the organisation. These are the nutrients of organisational culture. Any organisation that does not recognise the wide range of nutrients and embrace the impact they will have on change will not survive (Handy, 1999; Hall, 2005). The message is to be master of the direction the organisational culture takes (of the nutrients that are taken in and used) so that people with an investment in the organisation can feel, at least in part, in charge of the direction the organisation takes.

Thus organisational culture is something that is constantly evolving and reacting to changes around it. As such, it remains a matter of choice. It can be accepted, rejected or redesigned. However, if not attended to, it is still there. Invisible and all pervasive unless there is a move to try and feed it or change it appropriately. An organisation's vision may help set its direction and goals and it may be these that help it to find its way to the future. However, it is the organisation's values that help it get through the day-to-day activities and helps it thrive, survive or dive. It is the extent to which the managers and organisational brains – trust, realise that culture linked to values are the keys that help organisations make it home or, like the *Titanic*, hit an iceberg.

It is clear that an organisation's culture is influenced by many factors including economic, political, legal and technological elements, and by the context within which the organisation operates (Rytterstrom et al., 2013). In addition, the culture is influenced by the dominant values and behaviours of the majority of the organisation's members. These factors combined create the principal values, beliefs, norms and meanings that individuals infuse into the work they do. Scenario 7.1 provides an example of an organisation's culture being influenced by a set of dominant values.

SCENARIO 7.1   THE CADBURY STORY

The Cadbury's chocolate company was established in Birmingham, England in 1824, by John Cadbury. The business was developed further with his brother Benjamin and they moved to London. The company went into decline in the 1850s and John's sons, Richard and George, took over the business in 1861. In 1893 George bought 120 acres of land four miles from Birmingham and established the Bournville factory and estate. George developed the Bournville estate as a model village designed to give the company's workers improved living conditions and, significantly, for an English village there was no pub on the estate … but there was more to this company's organisational culture than the lack of a pub.

The Cadbury family were members of the Society of Friends, or Quakers, and in keeping with their beliefs they worked to end poverty and deprivation and initiate a number of social and industrial reforms. In this regard, John Cadbury's involvement with the Temperance Society influenced the initial direction of the business culture. From the start the business provided tea, coffee, cocoa and chocolate as an alternative to alcohol because John felt this was going some way to helping to alleviate some of the alcohol-related causes of poverty and deprivation among working people. He also incorporated some of these principles in his industrial relations philosophy.

However, it was John's sons, George and Richard, who proved to be the real business pioneers in industrial relations and employee welfare. As the company grew and prospered a series of novel – for Victorian Britain – working practices were implemented and additional facilities were provided for the workforce.

Cadbury was the first firm to introduce the Saturday half-day holiday (five and a half-day working week) and were pioneers in adopting the custom of closing the factory on Bank Holidays. In addition, a piecework system was initiated so that small rewards were given for punctuality and productivity. Also, educational needs were addressed and young employees were encouraged to attend night school and allowed to leave work an hour early twice a week.

When the new factory was built at Bournville it had many facilities which were unknown in Victorian times – separate gardens for men and women as well as extensive sports fields and women's and men's swimming pools, properly heated dressing rooms and kitchens for heating food. Sports facilities included football, hockey and cricket pitches; tennis and squash courts and a bowling green were also included.

To support social responsibility within the company, country outings and summer camps were organised. Special workers' fares were negotiated with the railway company and 16 houses were built for senior employees. Morning prayers and daily bible readings were begun in 1866 to preserve a family atmosphere and remained until the company grew too large to facilitate them.

George was also interested in improving the living conditions of working people. Thus the Bournville Village was built to provide affordable housing in pleasant surroundings for wage earners and to ensure that the environment around the Bournville factory did not fall into the hands of developers, so that their 'factory in a garden' could be maintained. The community was designed to be mixed in terms of both class and occupation, not just a village for Cadbury workers.

In 1900 George Cadbury handed over the land and houses to the Bournville Village Trust, with a charter to devote revenue to the extension of the estate and promote housing reform.

In the early days at Bournville, the Cadbury brothers ran the company as a family business (with the employees being thought of as part of the family) but as the business expanded a more formal management structure evolved that included workers committees to deal with issues affecting employees. Democratically elected works councils were set up in 1918, one for men and another for women, with equal numbers of management and worker representatives.

The councils were concerned with working conditions, health, safety, education, training and the social life of the factory and its workers. They remained unchanged for over half a century until 1965, when the men's and women's councils were merged. Today there is still employee participation in labour relations and negotiations.

(Continued)

(Continued)

It was not just the development of Dairy Milk chocolate (introduced in 1905 and their best seller by 1914) that helped build the fortunes of the Cadbury company. It was the original and ongoing commitment to their employees and their welfare that helped Cadbury stand apart from their competitors and to grow to become the second largest chocolate company in the world. Clearly, basing their company on a set of values that were evident in the actions of the Cadbury brothers and working on getting the organisational culture right has paid off in terms of profits and excellent products too.

The creation of an organisational culture is based on reinforcing the significance of key attributes, beliefs and values that build meaning and life into the organisation's culture. The central aspect of creating and maintaining a culture based on the key attributes, beliefs and values of an organisation relates to reinforcing and rewarding employees and members of the organisation who act on those values and beliefs and deliver performances consistent with the desired culture (Rytterstrom et al., 2013).

These cultures are also known as 'supportive cultures' (Luthans et al., 2008) and they are built upon the practice of energising and fostering the activity of the organisation's members (in all positions) to value and behave in ways that bolster and support the desired attributes, beliefs and values. Scenario 7.2 is an example of an organisation that is trying to follow this path to organisational change.

SCENARIO 7.2   THE NATIONAL HEALTH SERVICE CULTURE CHANGE STORY

In 2015, the UK Department of Health (DoH) released a document called *Culture Change in the NHS: Applying the Lessons of the Francis Inquiry* (DoH, 2015). In it, there is a recognition that while a culture change may have begun, sustaining that change will only be possible if doctors, nurses and front-line staff feel free to speak out if they have concerns. This has led to a deliberate drive to ensure the NHS is the 'most open and transparent (health) system in the world on key measures of patient safety and patient experiences' (DoH, 2015, p. 7).

To achieve this, a number of positive measures have been introduced. One involves a new legal duty, known as the 'duty of candour' (DoH, 2015). This places the responsibility on all NHS organisations to ensure that if anything does go wrong, patients and their relatives are informed immediately. Another initiative is the introduction of a 'name above the bed' system that will allow relatives and patients to know who is in charge of their care and who is accountable and responsible for their welfare. These few examples are evidence that change is taking place and, while only the beginning, a series of initiatives aimed at making the NHS more open and transparent are being fostered.

In addition, an unprecedented and bold effort has been made to capture feedback from patients, clients and their relatives using online and paper-based surveys, such as the 'friends and family test' (introduced in April 2013) to ask patients whether they would recommend their hospital to their friends and family (DoH, 2015). In this way feedback is used to bolster and support the positive steps health professionals are taking to build a refreshed culture with more focus on care and compassion.

The changes and initiatives in the example above are essential, because when organisational members see a lack of care and compassion for their welfare, for their skills, or for the contribution they could or do make, or if the feedback they provide is used as a stick to beat them. The message that is reinforced is that the organisation does not care for them or value them of their skills, and employees may feel they are seen simply as replaceable resources. This fosters a culture where suspicion, bullying, a lack of care and compassion and mistreatment is dominant and the net result is that the culture is one of suspicion, complacency and mistreatment (Francis, 2013; Rytterstrom et al., 2013).

In addition, all of the organisation's staff need to be trained and educated so that they can articulate their concerns when they speak up. The training should also include guidance and education about the pivotal place values and beliefs have when they are translated into actions (Stanley, 2011; DoH, 2015). If, indeed, leaders at all levels are central to shaping culture, then it is essential that leaders are supported and educated to provide effective, culturally appropriate leadership based on an organisation's foundational values. This again points to the place of Congruent Leadership and interprofessional working in helping foster a path to leadership for leaders at all levels, but most significantly for leaders who lack formal authority or titled positions.

This is the case for any industry, organisation, business or institution and the powerful place of an organisation's culture means that the net result is that the dominant culture is fostered and infused into the delivery of the organisation's product. If the product required is effective interprofessional communication, safe, holistic healthcare, and support and compassion for clients, then it will be of little surprise to find that quality healthcare, client support, interprofessional support networks and compassion fail to be consistently delivered if the dominant cultural narrative is negative, non-supportive of or non-responsive to a safety agenda.

If my business was a home gardening service and I wanted to build a reputation for having a reliable and dependable business but I was constantly late for appointments, failed to follow up on quotes or visit customers to undertake booked work, then it would be of little surprise if my business was soon considered the opposite to my intention and seen as unreliable and not dependable. Dominant values, as displayed through our actions, are translated into the service or product the organisation is responsible for.

ARTIFICIAL INTELLIGENCE AND CULTURE

Before going on with a discussion about the relationship of leadership and culture, I hope to digress a little to discuss the impact of the advent of artificial intelligence (AI) on culture. In recent times more and more organisations and industries are being influenced by the integration of AI into the workplace. For many years blue collar workplaces have been transformed by robotic machinery and the mechanisation of the workplace or production line. However, AI is now impacting directly on white-collar workplaces as industries and organisations seek to gather data and information on their workforce, their work and activity habits, and their productivity. On the surface it seems benign and, privacy concerns aside, there are strong arguments for the development of greater data-gathering on worker productivity.

However, it seems that the impact of this brave new world of data collection has not been tested in terms of its potential to change the face of an organisation's culture. If the manager is a machine, or if managers refer to data as the prime source of informa-tion to help make decisions about workplace relationships, productivity, worker interactions and worker social or peripheral activities, the nature (culture) of the work-place will be changed. If employers or organisations are able to monitor employees' time with clients, emotional responses to enquiries, effectiveness at set activities, time taken to undertake standard activities and a host of other activities or functions this will modify the way employees react to or engage with each other. In addition – and more importantly from a Congruent Leadership perspective – this may impact on how leadership is recognised or perceived within an organisation. If we are to be led by rigid targets, copious data or mechanistic approaches to productivity what messages will this send about the workplace culture, and who will staff or employees look to in order to role model the desired culture? What will leadership look like and how will leaders be recognised? Compliance and passivity may be seen as ideal features of the workplace with rewards related to outputs, targets and data sets being more valued than effective relationships, individuality, empowerment and creativity. It could be argued that AI is already impacting on productivity and organisational cultures and across the globe employees are already tied to data sets and production targets. However, for many workers in the Western world, greater monitoring and a data-driven workplace will dramatically change the shape of organisational cultures in ways that are yet to be determined. Workplaces, organisations and industries with a focus on the art and heart of their industry, profession or product may find that employees become conflicted when there is a move to embrace an output- and data-dominated focus, especially if this is perceived as a core shift in the organisational or professional cultural values.

CULTURE AND LEADERSHIP

For some time now, the health industry has recognised that to improve an organisa-tion's cultural practices they need to develop leaders and leadership that are focused on value-based approaches. Chalmers (2018, p. 9) said that 'nurse leaders have an absolute imperative to create a positive, accountable and transparent workplace.' In the UK, the DoH (2015) has specifically identified the need for leadership education and training (DoH, 2015, p. 16) in interprofessional practices, because 'the right leaders are critical in shaping culture.' As such they have recognised that with the right understanding of their values and how these impact on how they lead, greater impact on shaping organisational culture is likely. Reforms in government policy, organisational strategies and strategic documents (across the globe) have also called for improvements in organisational performance with many focusing on how leaders can better support interprofessional working and teamwork and a values-based organisational culture.

Where there is a failure to manage an organisation's culture, organisations need to deal, not with quality processes or quality assurance measures (although these may play a part) but with how to positively build or influence their organisation's cultural practices and how leaders within the organisations do this. The key to this link is the actions of the organisation towards their employees. As Congruent Leadership theory indicates, leaders are followed because they put into practice their values and beliefs. But these can be positive values as well as negative ones, so that staff follow the lead modelled by people identified as 'leaders' and those may be people the organisation may not recognise or realise are leaders. Therefore, if leaders (as identified by members of the organisation) are seen to act or treat staff in negative ways (not being listened to, mistreated, bullied, ignored or not valued for their skills or efforts) then it will not be a surprise if these behaviours are copied and repeated or seen as central to the organisation (because employees will recognise these behaviours as 'the way things are done around here'), especially if the leaders (however they are identified) are seen behaving in negative ways and are then promoted or rewarded.

The role of the senior executive is vital in setting the tone for an organisation's culture. However, as Hall (2005) indicates, most employees will see leaders at many levels and in this regard, it is the actions and behaviours of middle- or lower-level 'leaders' that are more likely to be dominant in setting an organisation's cultural tone.

Here is an example of how this may play out. Two police officers have a very different set of values that they apply to their job. One sees his police role as a warrior, a defender of liberty and a fighter of crime. His values are be tough, shoot first and ask questions second, be quick on the draw, look intimidating and show strength. Take no crap from anybody, see everyone, apart from close colleagues, as the enemy and recognise that the enemy is everywhere. If these values are taught or reinforced in the police officer's training or become a focus for the way they perform their job, then others will see them and recognise the officer as the 'warrior type'. The other police officer values community service, sees himself as a member of the community and, as such, seeks to be seen as a part of the community. He shows strength when needed but is also approachable and compassionate. He shows respect for others and listens as well as questions. He speaks quietly and confidently and he sees himself as a part of a wider social device for addressing the negative determinants of crime and social breakdown.

Each officer's different values mean that they will behave differently when faced with the various aspects of their job. They will be seen differently by their colleagues and co-workers, by their managers and by the public or their communities. They will use different language when making an arrest or interviewing someone at the police station. They will dress in ways that reflect their values (eyes hidden behind reflective sunglasses or not, uniforms laden with the tools of a warrior and covered in body armour or a uniform that is comfortable to wear while still showing the authority of the role and not the garb of one dressed for war). They will respond differently when confronted by various work situations. Occasionally, my everyday work brings me into contact with police services and I know which one of these officers I would feel safer with (and it is not the one with a big gun). However, would either of these officers have consciously thought about the values they employ or are they the product of the way they were trained or the environment in which they work? They have a choice of course, but they are both significantly influenced by the leaders they encounter and the specific set of values these leaders espouse.

Nurses that are 'task orientated' will behave differently to those that are 'client-centred' or 'person-centred'. As with the two police officers, their colleagues will see their different approach in the actions that support their different values. If I were a patient I would also know which set of values I should like applied to the care and attention I receive.

I teach nurses. The way I do it and the values that underpin the choice of things I say and roles I act out as a professional nurse very much impact on how student nurses learn and practise in the real world. If there is a disconnect between what I say and what I do the message is immediately weaker. If my actions role model a set of behaviours that are kind, compassionate, respectful and caring, then these are the messages students will receive most powerfully, and they will quickly see these behaviours as my values in action. The congruent message where our values and actions align becomes a very powerful tool for reinforcing the behaviour we want to enhance. It supports and builds the culture that is desired and helps shape the organisation or profession's culture.

HOW CONGRUENT LEADERS SHAPE CULTURE

Changing an organisation's culture is possible. However, it is only possible if it is understood that organisations have more than cultures. Indeed, they have cultures, structures and systems. Each is vital and without them organisations would crumble. The structure offers the skeleton of the organisation, helping to link responsibilities, roles, frameworks, facilities and equipment. Systems deal with how processes work and how people interact. Culture, however, is about the people, not cash, equipment, facilities or even product. Indeed, 'culture is *the* critical variable' in organisational success (Fitz-Enz, 1997).

Congruent Leadership is not directly focused on change. However, an organisation's culture can change when values and beliefs are challenged. Thus congruent leaders can influence change by acting in concert with their values and beliefs, especially if these offer an alternative to the current, dominant or prevailing culture. This is evident now with many organisations (even countries) being guided by leaders who demonstrate their values and beliefs and set the tone for the dominant culture of the organisation or country. When the leader has their values on display they are helping with the facilitation of change and therefore they become significant agents for change (even if they don't know it or even if the behaviours or actions are negative). The result is that the change they institute can be very powerful. As suggested in Chapter 4:

- *Vision* is about where an organisation is going ... and what an organisation is doing.
- *Values* are about how an organisation is doing what it is doing ... values drive decisions and become the foundations of the culture (the underlying assumptions), contributing to the design and function of the operating system and the organisation's structure.

As such, establishing a values-based culture further underpins the organisation's vision. With values and beliefs also linking to a person's emotional and relationship networks, congruent leaders are in positions to influence and build powerful and lasting organisational cultures.

Leaders are therefore required to shape culture by taking responsibility for where they sit within an organisation and recognising their behaviours and actions will be seen, followed and copied, even if the organisational hierarchy is unable to witness the impact they are having. Bickhoff (2018, p. 10) suggests this can be done 'one shift at a time' if front-line nurses (and other professional staff) 'decide to be the change they want to see on their ward.' This points the way, but there are a number of other ways leaders can foster organisational change. Hall (2005) suggested the following activities that I have expanded upon:

- Leaders need to become models of the culture or 'champions of culture'. The research that forms the basis of the theory of Congruent Leadership identified that being a role model was central to how shopfloor, coalface, bedside or non-hierarchical leaders were recognised.
- Leaders need to remain visible in their 'modelling role'. Being visible was another key attribute of this type of leadership and meant that congruent leaders were recognised as visible, approachable and present.
- Leaders need to ensure other senior staff support and also model the desired culture (staff at all levels in an organisation see different people as 'senior leaders' depending on where they are placed and who they interact with). In this

regard mid-level and even lower-level leaders/managers are vital. This is the case for all types of industry or organisation. Leaders are identified and recognised at all levels of an organisation and significantly so. They may even be less likely to be seen at senior management levels or at the door of people in positions of control (because they may not be seen actually leading or putting in place their values). If they are not seen applying their values then there is the potential for a lack of visibility to be regarded as the expression of values that negates support, shows a lack of interest in the welfare or well-being of employees and staff. The net result may be a contribution to a culture of 'us and them' that may kill off an institution or organisation.

- Leaders need to develop personal ownership and responsibility for their behaviour and how it will impact on others or be seen by others. This suggests that leaders cannot just 'talk the talk'. They need to be seen to 'live' their values and beliefs and put these into action – and not in a superficial or cursory way. Actions need to be meaningful. As an example of this I once worked at an organisation where the management felt that they would show their appreciation of the staff by adding a Mars Bar to the pay slips of all employees. The net result was not what had been anticipated. A mass of discontent spread through the organisation as staff interpreted the gesture as implying that management felt all their hard work was worth only as much as a small chocolate bar.

- Leaders need to employ personal communication approaches (avoid email where possible), speak with people, establish communication approaches that support individual approaches to people. This supports the attributes of congruent leaders who use excellent communication skills and lead by their actions rather than just what they say they will do.

- Leaders need to repeat messages in a number of ways to ensure they are received consistently and effectively. This again rests on the congruent leader's ability to use excellent communication skills, the key to establishing personal and meaningful communication and having others see the leader's values in action, to build respect and trustworthiness and to keep communication clear with open interpersonal skills. To achieve this ask yourself:

  o   Can people believe what I am saying?
  o   Do I listen to others' concerns?
  o   Are my intentions and actions clear and consistent?
  o   Are my actions consistent (congruent) with my values?
  o   Do I say and do what I mean?
  o   Do I know what my values are and are these expressed in my actions?

In addition, Garvin and Roberto (2005) suggest that effective leaders (congruent leaders) provide opportunities for employees to practise desired behaviours repeatedly while personally modelling new ways of working and providing coaching and support. In this way effective congruent leaders explicitly reinforce their own and (hopefully) the organisation's values on a consistent basis, using actions to back up their words.

In order to establish lasting cultural change employees and staff need to be rewarded for actions that support and promote any new or desirable ways of operating. Appropriate rewards will send clear messages about the desired culture (more on this is offered in Chapter 8). How these behaviours are rewarded is also important with the more effective rewards producing the more rapid and lasting change. Rafferty et al. (2015) add, after interviewing a number of staff in the UK, that NHS staff suggested that their commitment, productivity and engagement were strongly linked to four themes essential for them to feel part of a positive work culture. They said they needed:

- the resources to deliver their job;
- the support to do a good job;
- a worthwhile job that offers the chance to develop;
- the opportunity to improve teamworking.

There is considerable evidence to support the conclusion that monetary rewards or general awards are not rated highly. Pink (2009) suggests there are three factors that lead people to perform better and increase their personal satisfaction at work. Firstly, people are motivated by mastery (our urge to get better at things); secondly, by autonomy (a desire to be self-directed); and thirdly, by purpose (a desire to find meaning in the things we do) (Pink, 2009). Indeed Pink (2009) is of the view that the more the profit motive becomes detached from the purpose motive, the more bad things happen. So that congruent leaders who are able to link their values and beliefs to their actions may find this is a more effective motivator for why leaders may be more effective in leading and changing organisational culture.

The following are offered as a guide to organisational change from a values-based leadership perspective. These are:

- *Prevent problems.* Employ transparency, acknowledge issues and respond to mistakes by recognising that more may need to be done.
- *Promote more freedom of speech and autonomy.* Most people in work want their organisations to do well. They want to feel they are part of the mechanisms for making the business grow or making the company stronger, better or more well-recognised.
- *Detect problems quickly and do something about them.* Deal with complaints appropriately, seeking relevant feedback and engage or connect with a wider range of service users in the delivery and consultation about the service or industry.
- *Address any issues of sexual harassment or employee-to-employee bullying promptly and resolutely.* Be clear about behavioural expectations from the start, at the orientation or induction of new staff, and remind current or long-term staff what is and is not appropriate. Ensure everyone knows the processes for how to report and deal with inappropriate behaviours and what the consequences are for employees who fail to meet the standards expected.

- *Take action promptly and retain a robust process for accountability.* This implies that the people who are accountable ensure that what is meant to happen does happen. Employ inspections, ratings, clear lines of accountability and measures to ensure accountabilities are understood and acted upon.
- *Move away from a culture of blame.* Doing so will reduce risk, increase safety and promote greater employee engagement.
- *Ensure staff are trained and motivated.* This involves developing leadership skills and practices in keeping with a culture based on values and beliefs and interprofessional teamworking. It also means that all members of the organisation should be aware of the 'right values' (or the ones promoted by the organisation).
- *Finally, it is incumbent on the organisation to support staff.* As Dixon-Woods et al. (2013) indicate, there is a close relationship between the well-being of staff and the success of an organisation and its profitability.

The key to changing an organisation's culture lies in changing and reinforcing desired behaviour and positively supporting the message about the organisation's desired values. Leaders then need to role model the desired values in what they do (not just what they say) and encourage everyone to play their part in shaping the organisation's culture. Then, leaders need to invite participation, ownership and commitment from colleagues and team members. It is often said 'That which we create, we cherish.' You may recall that the wolf we feed will win. Therefore lasting change is based upon using appropriate rewards to reinforce desired behaviours and values. From this standpoint, organisations will then establish respect, grow trust and communicate more effectively (with the staff, employees, students, clients, teachers, drivers, packers, sales assistants, stakeholders, etc.). Once the values are clear and the organisation knows what underpins its foundations then the organisation's vision, strategic plan and way forward can be established.

EXAMPLES OF CONGRUENT LEADERS

Offering a more modern and organisational example of Congruent Leadership are Nicholas Marchesi and Lucas Patchett, school friends who in 2014 realised that homeless Australians needed an opportunity to have clean clothes, something most people take for granted. They decided to do something about it. They obtained a van, took out the interior and bolted a washing machine and dryer inside. It took some time to get the logistics right but before long they were providing the world's first mobile laundry for homeless people sleeping rough in Brisbane, on Australia's east coast. In this simple way, Orange Sky laundry was born.

Nicholas and Lucas begged, borrowed and stole (only the water I think) and grew the service they provided from the one van, called 'Suddsy', to a fleet of vans operated by over 600 volunteers across Australia, washing an estimated 7.2 tonnes of laundry for homeless people each week. In 2016 they were jointly awarded the

Young Australian of the Year Award and were secured a place as leading members of a company based fundamentally on their values. However, they are very clear that while the vans and volunteers provide a laundry service (and they have since expanded to offer a hair cutting service) this is only the 'vehicle' to support their main value, which is connecting with the people they meet on the streets and in the parks. Their initial aim was to improve hygiene standards and restore dignity to people doing it; however, they stumbled on something much bigger and more significant – the power of a conversation. The need they eventually saw being over-looked may have been a basic one of hygiene, but the laundry service is funda-mentally an opportunity to connect with and spend time with people who are commonly on the fringes of society. This is what Nicholas and Lucas believe the laundry service is really about;

> Orange Sky Laundry is a catalyst for conversation. In the one-hour time it takes to wash and dry someone's clothes there is absolutely nothing to do but sit down on one of our 6 orange chairs and have a positive and genuine conversation

Source: Orange Sky Australia

Setting up a philanthropic and charitable service like Orange Sky takes courage and in their case a degree of naivety that provided the 'never say give up' spirit the venture needed. Orange Sky is based on their respect for all people, for addressing basic human needs and is very strongly about being empathetic and connecting with a vulnerable and commonly disadvantaged group. There was no profit motive and it required significant determination, resilience and perseverance. Their passion for promoting and growing the service makes it clear that they are both congruent leaders, leading with their values on show for others to recognise and follow.

Much of what I have read about Barack Obama (President of the USA between 2009 and 2016) points towards him being a congruent leader. While there are many examples of his leadership style that could be cited in support of a range of leader-ship theories, I will use just one example of Barack Obama as a congruent leader in action.

In July 2009, a Harvard University professor called Henry Gates Jr returned home from a trip to China only to find the front door to his home jammed shut. He and his driver forced the door open and a passing witness, thinking they were breaking in reported the event to the police. Police responded and determined quickly that it was Gates' own home, but Gates became upset at the attitude of the police and one of the attending officers (Sgt James Crowley) arrested Gates for disorderly conduct. The specific events leading to the arrest are still unclear, but the international media picked up on the story and described it as an example of a racially motivated arrest or an example of racial profiling by the police.

Obama offered comments to the media on the issue (that he later regretted) and although the charges were dropped a week later, Obama, seeking to build some-thing positive from the event invited Gates and Crowley and the Vice-President

(Joe Biden) to the White House garden for a discussion with him over a beer. The event became known as the 'beer summit' and while it seems limited agreement was reached, the conversation was described as 'cordial and positive' by Crowley, who added that they all 'agreed to look forward rather than backward'. Obama said, 'I have always believed that what brings us together is stronger than what pulls us apart. I am confident that has happened here tonight, and I am hopeful that all of us are able to draw this positive lesson from this episode.' Obama used the event and publicity it generated as a 'teachable moment' about tolerance and the power of personal connection. As a congruent leader, Obama was able to recognise his mistake, invite discussion and reach out to bring people together. As President, he was not aloof or too removed from vital issues of public concern, and his personal involvement in the discussion allowed others to see he valued conversation and discourse over rhetoric and soundbite or doing nothing.

There is one other example of a congruent leader in this chapter. She is a young girl called Malala Yousafzai. She was born in 1997 and grew up in the Swat Valley in Northwest Pakistan. Eager to promote better education for girls and women in Pakistan she spoke out in protest about Taliban restrictions on girls being educated. Between the ages of 11 and 12 Malala wrote a 'blog' detailing her life under the Taliban and this brought her to the attention of the international community. In 2009 the *New York Times* made a documentary about her life and she was recognised as an advocate for human rights and especially regarded for speaking out against educational restrictions for girls in Pakistan. Sadly, in 2012 she and two other girls were attacked in an attempted assassination attempt while they travelled home on a bus. Critically injured after being shot in the head, Malala was eventually transferred to the Queen Elizabeth Hospital in Birmingham in the UK.

The attempt on her life initiated worldwide support and even with the Taliban professing to continue to target her she set up a non-profit organisation and co-authored a book *I Am Malala* with the aim of continuing to speak out against the repression of women and for greater access to education for young women and girls. In 2015 Malala was awarded, as a co-recipient, the 2014 Nobel Peace Prize. In her short life Malala has been recognised as one of the most influential people globally and while she is yet to return to her home province in the Swat Valley, Malala is recognised as a courageous and passionate advocate for the rights of women and girls. She is currently studying in Oxford, UK and in spite of the fatwa against her she continues to speak out and remains a prominent activist for a cause that almost cost her her life. Malala is a congruent leader seeking the education she advocates for others and showing the way by doing what she believes is the right thing to do. Malala is an important leader who has held on tightly to her ambition to be educated and to show others the way with her values on show.

CHAPTER SUMMARY

Organisational culture describes the pattern of beliefs, values and behaviours that have evolved within organisations that leads members of the organisation (and others) to come to terms with how things are done within it. While there are different types of organisational culture and ways to explore or understand various levels of their culture, organisational culture is predominantly people focused. As such, the key to changing or building an organisation's culture lies in changing and reinforcing the behaviour and values of the people within the institution. This can be achieved with displays, rewards or prompts for the desired values or behaviours that show how the organisation is to be recognised. Leaders at all levels of an organisation are vital for this to be achieved. It is also proposed that Congruent Leadership theory strongly supports links between culture, values, beliefs and leadership, and as such it is leaders who are able to role model the desired behaviours or values that will support an organisation's cultural growth and development or cement the cultural fingerprint of an organisation. The next chapter explores how Congruent Leadership may be applied in the workplace in support of reinforcing organisational culture.

8

THE APPLICATION OF CONGRUENT LEADERSHIP IN THE WORKPLACE

'It's not hard to make decisions when you know what your values are.'

Roy Disney, American businessman

INTRODUCTION

This chapter considers ways organisations and individuals can apply Congruent Leadership to enhance their leadership potential and bring about positive change in their workplace and professional lives. The chapter too concludes by exploring further examples of congruent leaders and describing leaders who lead by matching their values and beliefs with their actions.

BE CLEAR ABOUT YOUR OWN VALUES

Be clear about your own values. This may sound self-evident. We all have values and these are commonly expressed consciously or unconsciously every day in the things we do and the things we say. However, do we really ever or often take stock of what they are? I suggest that, in general, we do not. If we are faced with a conscious opportunity to express or think about our values we may consider them, for example when writing wedding vows, when completing a dating site profile, if applying for a new job or if faced with a major life changing event such as a near-death experience or another person's death or near-death experience. However, most of the time, most of us do not live lives where we consciously take account of or frame our lives, particularly our work lives, through the lens of our values.

There are some people who might do so more commonly such as religious practitioners, e.g. monks, nuns, rabbis, imams, priests, pastors to name a few. These are people you might expect to base their lives on a set of values aligned with the religion's teachings or the values appropriate to their understanding of the religious principles they follow. Political leaders do this too (or I would hope they do) as they align themselves with a political party's core values or as they apply their personal values in the interests they take or causes they support. However, what Congruent Leadership stresses is that leaders are followed because others recognise the leader's values in the things they do and are drawn to follow them because of this congruence. Many congruent leaders do not realise they are being followed for this reason and as such it is not common for leaders to be cognisant or aware of the values they display.

ACTIVITY 8.1   REFLECTIVE EXERCISE

Take time to reflect on what you think are fundamental values you hold as important, even vital, to you and specifically through the performance or in the act of your work.

This can take the form of a reflection, where I would encourage you to think about your personal or individual values. Take time to write them down.

Therefore, the first practical suggestion offered here is for leaders or potential leaders (everyone really) to be aware of their own values. Think about the words you have used. It may be worth discussing the list with someone who you trust and seek feedback on how honest and realistic you have been. It need not be an extensive list. You should, however, aim for a list of meaningful words for you. Does the list resonate with things you value firmly? When it comes to values the idea is to stand like a rock. It is only in matters of fashion that we should go with the flow. Does your list capture those things that you would stand firmly and resolutely by?

It may be difficult to make a list based on your personal or individual values. If so, focus on your professional or workplace values. In many cases they may overlap. Reflect again and make a separate list. Think carefully about the words you use and what they mean. I am a nurse, I value, kindness, compassion, care, honesty and integrity, authenticity and respect for others. I also value high-quality care and the application of competence, skills and knowledge. I would hope that my colleagues hold the same values, but they may not or they may have others on their list. They may also describe the same or similar things in different ways. Talk with your colleagues or workmates about your list and see if they agree or disagree. If yours is a list of personal values, talk with your partner, wife, husband, children, other relatives or friends. What are their values? Are they the same? Having talked to them, are you more or less confident in the words on your list? Has your list been challenged? Once you have had the conversation, do you feel able to defend or stand by your words or are you questioning your values?

If I worked in a bank or an insurance company I might hold different values. I would hope honesty and integrity would remain, but my focus may be more on quality service or prompt service or selling appropriate products to the right people. Or my values might be on making sure the maximum profit is extracted from customers regardless of their circumstances. I was in a bank recently and picked up a *Code of Banking Practice* (Australian Bankers Association, 2013). It provided over 40 pages of information and even included a section on 'Our commitments to you', but at no point did it make clear what their values were. Some very high-profile banks that sign up to and distribute this booklet to their customers have been exposed as having dubious practices, where it seems as if their values were on making a maximum profit, if not at the expense of their customers, certainly it seems with little regard for the service customers receive or even the impact of their practices on the community or the environment or on wider ethical practices.

Knowing your personal, individual values or recognising your professional or workplace values is important because they may be in conflict with your employer's values or with those of the people you work with. Knowing where your values are in relation to your employer or the people you work with will allow you to find your place in an organisation or workplace and will either enhance or limit the potential for conflict. I have left a few jobs I have had over the years, not because the pay was poor or the location was inappropriate or the trip to work was long and stressful, but because I didn't feel I was able to be who I really was when I was at work. This led to a state of moral distress that kept me awake at night and worried when at work. The John Hopkins Nursing publication (2017) suggested that moral distress could be a threat to nurse retention. It plagues significant numbers of nurses and many other healthcare professionals. Nurses, they suggested, may not be able to fulfil their nursing obligations to their patients due to intractable value conflicts, poor staffing policies, ineffective communication, lack of teamwork, organisational oversights and a general pressure on the healthcare system undermining the integrity and well-being of staff. From my own experiences, I was sometimes asked to do things that just felt wrong or that I felt conflicted with my values, either as a person or a professional, or I found myself working with people (often in power) who expressed or held values that I found unconscionable. Has this ever happened to you?

I was once an acting hospital manager and was asked by the organisation's leadership to close a ward in one month. I agree that sometimes we have to make hard decisions. I understood this part of my job. The closure was a short-term fix for a critical financial crisis. It made some sense as the organisation's finances really were in a dire state but it would mean a reduction of services to a specific group of clients. The staff on the ward were mostly women and a significant majority were married to or in relationships with men who had until recently worked in the local car industry, which had collapsed putting these men out of work. The idea that we would simply close a ward as the only response to the financial crisis showed (in my view) a lack of managerial imagination. I felt compromised as I was instructed to undertake the closure in a very short time. The local community, through the press and at public meetings, were outraged and I had every sympathy with their views and the distress of the staff. I, however, was the face of the closure and became at once the instrument of their distress and the target for their anger.

I worked very hard to try and manage the situation. I opened regular weekly communication sessions with all hospital staff, as the closure impacted in one way or another on everyone. I sought to find staff who were able and willing to take early retirement or redundancy packages. Fortunately, there were a handful of staff who welcomed the opportunity to finish work. I found a few staff who wanted to undertake more training and these were supported to take on further study and I helped with study leave packages. A few staff could be moved to other wards and we managed to negotiate for others to move to jobs at affiliated institutions. No one was sacked. Everyone was consulted and given choices, and in most cases people were cared for and supported and able to move to suitable and appropriate work or on to retirement. The client group lost out the most. Many now had to travel further for care and the extra pressure put on the other areas of the hospital meant that the general services were more stretched and harder to manage.

I managed the closure well, in respect of my not having to compromise my own values or the core values of the organisation as they related to treating patients and staff with care, compassion and respect. I took more than the allocated month (I took two), as I used time to address the many staff and client concerns. In spite of my best efforts I was not asked to apply for the permanent position. Caring for people (staff and clients) and making sure that they were communicated with clearly, dealt with respectfully and given choices were not (it turned out) the organisation's dominant values. They did value reducing costs and I had taken too long. I returned to my substantive post and smartly started looking for another place to work. At the time I hadn't realised that the internal conflict I felt about doing what I thought was the right thing (for the staff and clients) as opposed to doing what the organisation wanted was a clash of values. I doubt the organisation thought about this issue in this way either. I do contest, however, that if they had really considered their values prior to making the decision to close the ward, they may have seen or been driven to find a more reasonable and productive solution to their financial crisis or have managed the situation differently and, possibly, more positively. It is possible that a lack of focus on values contributed to them being in the dire financial state they were in in the first place.

Therefore being clear about your own values matters, firstly so you can support and live them, but also so you can choose to be with or foster relationships with people that share your values or perhaps better understand people whose values may differ. In addition, you can recognise if your values bring you into conflict with what you feel is important to you.

BE CLEAR ABOUT YOUR ORGANISATION'S VALUES

If an employer is reading this, it is not enough to recognise your own personal values. I would strongly advocate for every organisation to reflect, discuss, meet and struggle to know what their organisational values really are, to test these out, to print them out, to sound them out. Putting them on a poster and pinning it to a tearoom wall is not enough. I would recommend painting them in large bold letters in prominent places about the organisation. Narrabri Hospital in Western NSW have their values painted in big white letters just inside the main foyer. I was there to interview staff about their understanding of leadership and each person I spoke with was able to talk about their connection to the hospital's values. There was no ambiguity about what the organisation's values were and staff spoke about everyone modelling the values painted on the wall.

Once upon a time, organisations and even families had mottos. The high school I went to had one. It was and remains 'Una Omnibus Scholar'. As students we speculated over what it meant – 'One student came to school by bus' perhaps? Instead it really meant something like 'learning for all'. To an extent this captured a hint of the school's values; however, a motto doesn't go far enough. Usually more than one theme is captured in a set of values. It is not enough to claim to have values, or to paint them on a wall, or boast of a motto, or put the words on a poster. Identify them, please do, but values only come to life if lived.

I have previously mentioned the values of the North American energy company Enron and clearly they did not relate to the actions or practice of the company. In the following section I will outline a number of other organisations' values to see what they might say about these institutions.

FROM THE OLYMPIC MOVEMENT

Olympism is a philosophy of life, exalting and combining in a balanced whole the qualities of body, will and mind. Blending sport with culture and education, olympism seeks to create a way of life based on the joy found in effort, the educational value of good example and respect for universal fundamental ethical principles.

International Olympic Movement

They add that their goal is 'to contribute to building a peaceful and better world by educating youth through sport practised without discrimination of any kind and in the Olympic spirit, which requires mutual understanding with a spirit of friendship, solidarity and fair play.'

FROM ST JOHN OF GOD HOSPITAL IN PERTH, WA

'For a short time I worked at this hospital in Perth and during the two-day orientation the five key values of the hospital were front and centre as myself and other new staff were introduced to what was expected from staff. The five values were: Justice, Excellence, Hospitality, Respect and Compassion. The values of St John of God healthcare were intended to influence how caregivers delivered services throughout the organisation.'

FROM THE WORLD BANK

The World Bank has no values statements on its web page, but it does offer two 'goals': 'To end extreme poverty and promote shared prosperity in a sustainable way' (http://www.worldbank.org/, accessed on 3 February 2018). As discussed in Chapter 4, vision and values are not the same thing and goals, while an excellent statement of an aspiration, may not reflect the values an organisation will apply in reaching their goals.

FROM AMAZON

Amazon has an interesting take on their values. They suggest that 'Whether you are an individual contributor or the manager of a large team, you are an Amazon leader. These are our leadership principles and every Amazonian is guided by these principles.' Their 'principles' are also their core values:

- Customer obsession
- Ownership
- Invent and Simplify
- Are right, a lot
- Hire and develop the best
- Insist on the highest standards
- Think big
- Bias for action
- Frugality
- Vocally self-critical

- Earn trust of others
- Dive deep
- Have backbone; disagree and commit
- Deliver results

They add that their 'mission statement is also their vision.' Their 'vision is to be earth's most customer centric company; to build a place where people can come to find and discover anything they might want to buy online.' Pretty impressive, as they have linked the concept that if leadership is everyone's business, then everyone will be invested in their business (http://www.theleadermaker.com/core-values-amazon-com/, accessed on 3 February 2018). There may, however, be questions about the effectiveness with which Amazon hits these value targets.

FROM BHP

Broken Hill Proprietary Company (BHP), a large Australian mineral company, has a simple statement that describes their 'Approach'. In it they state: 'Wherever we operate in the world, we strive to work with integrity – doing what is right and doing what we say we will do.' They elaborate on this and suggest that they are about 'working with integrity', adding 'we are fully committed to working with integrity and our Code of Business Conduct. Like safety, working with integrity – doing what is right and doing what we say we will do – should be the starting point for everything we do. We care as much about how results are achieved as we do about the results themselves' (www.bhp.com/our-approach/operating-with-integrity, accessed on 3 February 2018).

Values have to be lived out as well as be on display and applied constantly and vividly. To apply values consistently organisations and even departments within them need to reflect, think, discuss, debate and agree on the values they hold or wish to be associated with. The process for this can be far more complex than simply having the board or senior staff meet to write down their values for other staff to follow. The process itself, if shared with staff, can be a gesture of collaboration and a lived value of engagement and cooperation. However, this will only occur if indeed these are values the organisation hold. If the board of directors or senior staff do indeed stipulate a set of values without consultation, this is also modelling a set of values that negates cooperation, open communication and engagement with staff or employees. This too influences the organisation's culture and sets the tone for how staff in the organisation interact.

I have worked for a number of organisations where they have undergone values-building or values-documenting activities. In some organisations these activities felt like and proved to be simple lip service to the consultation process and management were simply ticking an organisational or industry accreditation box. In the end the values were meaningless to most staff and were relegated to framed lists on hallway walls or on notice boards by the lift. The process is not just about capturing the list of values but translating them into the actions of leaders and staff within and across the organisation. As such, the process of generating the values and living them out are indeed very complex. Role modelling values achieves far more than a list on a wall. However, the values themselves need to be considered, discussed and agreed to so that they can be universally applied, through all strata of an organisation. Making them known and claiming them is only the first step.

ROLE MODEL YOUR VALUES

To a large part this is the core of how Congruent Leadership works. Deciding how to behave and how you will undertake to treat people (patients, clients, customers, colleagues, staff or workmates) will occur by conscious choice or by subconscious habit. Our actions do not lie. Some people may be good actors, but pretending to hold one set of values and acting these out when actually holding another set is a very difficult act to maintain. Ultimately, we are all seen for the values we genuinely hold. This is true of both people and organisations. The strength of congruence is in matching our values and beliefs with our actions. If the message sent and received lacks ambiguity it will make a powerful point, even if you are not aware of the match between the two.

Visibility is a key feature of role modelling. From an organisational perspective, leaders need to be seen applying themselves and their actions to the values of the organisation. This will not occur if the leaders and managers or people charged with leading at a range of levels are not seen. General Hamilton, who was in command of the British and Australian forces at Gallipoli during the First World War, was criticised because he rarely set foot on the Gallipoli peninsula and few of the troops saw him. In general, First World War senior officers were considered from much the same critical perspective. Many failed to appreciate trench warfare and few officers suffered as the men did. Alexander the Great may have been inclined to be too eager to role model the behaviours he expected of his troops on the battlefield and he put his life on the line in the same way he expected his troops to. Consequently, many saw his exploits, and were encouraged and motivated by them. Alexander the Great could never be criticised for not role modelling the values he saw as vital for military success.

Who people see as the leader matters because in all organisations people rarely meet or work closely with very senior managers. Richard Branson (the head of the Virgin Group of organisations, business magnate, investor and philanthropist) may offer an example of a modern industrial or business leader who is visible in the running of his businesses. Andrew Forrest – or 'Twiggy' as he is sometimes known – may be another. His former leadership of the Fortescue Metals Group ensured that almost every employee knew him by sight and recognised his values through his down-to-earth style and generous support for a range of social policy issues and Indigenous cultural projects.

Both Richard Branson and Andrew Forrest may be exceptions. Most high-level business leaders are recognised only because their photo is in the introduction of the annual report, or because they appear periodically at local social functions or philanthropic events. As such, most employees and staff look to leaders they see frequently or on a daily basis to role model the organisation's or their own values.

It is no use for senior managers to role model the values they hope to support or promote if only a small percentage of the workforce see the behaviour. Not being seen in action means that myths and stories build that may or may not put the leader in a positive or negative light. Depending on a cascade approach to the delivery of values in action is a risky move. In effect the leader or senior manager is passing on responsibility to others to behave and display their values on their behalf. The risk of course is that not everyone else will share or role model the values senior managers hope to serve, especially if these have not been made explicit or if the de facto leaders are unaware of this role, are poor communicators or take it upon themselves to role model their own set of values (positive or negative).

In the past, monthly or weekly newsletters or annual reports have been used to communicate values or organisational stories that support or promote values. With greater electronic resources for sharing information, senior leaders should be able to find ways to 'get their message' out to all staff and bolster their visibility as they role model the desired organisational values. However, the strongest message is the presence of a leader acting out their personal or organisational values in the vicinity of the people they are hoping to influence or lead.

ROUNDING (WALKING THE WALK)

A specific approach to role modelling is the practice of 'rounding'. This practice is where leaders and/or managers take time to visit the workplace and work location of employees on a regular and consistent basis. This is becoming more and more common in the health sector. This is not to check up on employees or staff, or to catch people not doing their work, but to be seen and to be present on the shop floor, on the ward, in the office, in the corridors of the school or at the coalface. It permits direct communication about key issues, such as any safety or resource concerns. It allows a first-hand observation of working conditions or the challenges employees may be facing. It lets the manager or leader be seen and it facilitates greater appreciation by each party of the other's work role. It need not take a long time, but it does take time. It cannot be delegated, because this negates the impact of the act of being visible.

It may result in genuine opportunities to introduce innovation, offset potential problems or threats to the organisation and stimulate discussions about new or better ways to reduce risks or improve working conditions or productivity. At the very least it will allow staff and employees to get to know the person who manages or leads them at work. It is like an open-door policy, but instead of people coming to the manager, the manager/leader goes to the staff/employee. It comes with risks. Not all managers want to get to know their staff. Not all managers want to be on 'friendly' terms with the people they manage. However, in order to build a more collaborative culture or support greater communication, and to reduce safety risks and engage employees with the core organisational culture and values, it may be that by taking on the attributes of a congruent leader, success is more likely. In this way leaders are visible, role modelling the values they wish to support or promote. Nothing works more effectively than a personal approach and nothing of worth can be achieved without making the effort to be present and stand alongside others, even for only a short time each month or each week. It is akin to the principle of the 'undercover boss' (a reality TV show where the 'boss' takes on a disguise and mixes with various employees for a short time to get a feel for the 'shopfloor' level activity of their company), but without the 'undercover' aspect.

COME TOGETHER

Finding ways to meet at or outside of work will help build a set of common values. It also limits isolation and builds a sense of community and collaboration. This is important for professional groups to ensure they build their identity, but it is also vital that there is interprofessional and cross-disciplinary meetings and social events so that each can also recognise the value of diversity and difference and see that indeed, they commonly share the same values. Celebrating differences is important, but so too is being able to recognise that we are part of a collective whole, accepted and supported. Culture, teamwork, partnerships and collaboration grow from shared emotional events. Coming together also implies a recognition of and celebration of teamworking.

GIVING VOICE TO VALUES

Knowing your values, or knowing your organisation's values and then displaying them in action, visibly in our personal life or at work, matters in terms of creating powerful leadership. This next step is about encouraging others to discover and recognise their values. Our values are ours. The organisation's values are commonly developed and outlined by others, but even if they are not, and if we are invited to contribute to or build an organisation's values, many people may not feel their values matter. They may not make the connection between them and their place in an organisation, or the place of values in shaping their place in the many relationships they have, including with their employer.

This step in the application of Congruent Leadership is about encouraging or asking others to consider their values and the place they have in their personal or work lives. I am often surprised to hear that discussing values is seen as a weakness and/or an irrelevance. This perspective is commonly an expression of insecurity and it will only undermine efforts to genuinely build insight into where people and organisations stand and what they see as important. Knowing about and talking about where we stand matters, as much as being aware of what matters. If values are not discussed or given voice, it is probably because they are not being acted upon. Values pinned to a tearoom wall and ignored or not acted upon are as useful as a flag pole with no rope to hoist the flag. Flags, like values, only matter when they are unfurled and seen flying.

REWARD DESIRABLE VALUES

A powerful tool for promoting the expression of desired values in an organisation is to reward the expression or performance (action) of the values seen as core to the organisation. Appropriate rewards will send clear and unambiguous messages about the values that are significant in each organisation. These do not have to be monetary rewards – in fact these often work in an inverse way and neither support key values nor promote greater actions in line with values. The key to this type of reward and recognition is generally personal recognition and may even be informal in nature. Again, this requires that the leader/manager is visible and present so that they are able to recognise the expression of the desired values in action.

If an employee or member of staff is recognised for behaving in a way that supports or complements the organisation's values the leader or manager could comment on this directly to the staff member. 'Hi, Bill, I overheard your conversation with that customer who was making a complaint. You were patient and clear, explaining our policies and processes well. You took time to listen, were respectful and you offered them an excellent solution. Thank you, I really appreciate the care you took with them.' This indicates the specific behaviours that were noted and why they were appropriate and it implies they were in line with the organisation's values and provides a personal expression of gratitude from a manager/leader. Most staff and employees will respond positively to this type of feedback. It will further support an organisational culture that builds on the organisation's core values. Personal positive feedback is generally very powerful, especially if offered with sincerity and in a genuine way. This message could be sent in an email, but the power of the role modelling opportunity and the personal aspect of the message is diminished significantly. Email is not a great tool for supporting staff rewards (Hall, 2005).

Hall (2005) also suggested other rewards that may be appropriate, including offering informal feedback, opportunities for further professional development or recognition at team or group events. Staff could also be recognised with specific projects that attract greater responsibility and promotion opportunities, as long as they are not perceived as 'more work' or 'harder work' as this is seldom seen as a reward. Time to work on personal projects or opportunities for personal study and additional leave are also powerful motivators and act as great rewards. In some organisations staff are given 'stock options' or a percentage of any profits generated from an innovation they have developed. In some industries holidays and weekend breaks are used as rewards and while these all work well, they each have the potential to become the object of the work effort and not the satisfaction of working towards the values of the organisation.

What is really clear as a demotivator is when staff or employees who are seen by many other staff as shirkers or bullies or incompetent are rewarded with less work, special projects or promotions. The message in these cases is that poor performance and incompetence is rewarded and this acts as a direct demotivator for staff and employees who do the right thing and are overlooked or ignored. Inequity in the work place is a motivation killer. Ultimately, good staff who feel unfairly treated will leave and the organisation will ring to the hollow bell of incompetence and bias.

DEAL WITH POOR BEHAVIOUR

Call discrimination, harassment and bullying for what it is. Support robust management and human resource interventions for inappropriate behaviours. Report breaches of appropriate employee behaviour and conduct. Support clear guidelines or policies for dealing with poor behaviour. Hold yourself and others to a higher standard that acknowledges when breaches have occurred, and have the courage to confront colleagues who hold others in contempt and bully or harass.

SEEK OUT DIVERSITY

While it is important to feel secure within a workplace culture, sometimes seeking new perspectives and looking at the world from a different angle is vital. Seeking and supporting diversity, testing the borders of our values is occasionally an important step for ensuring we can be flexible when needed and open to change. Being able to accommodate diversity may lead to new ideas or new ways to solve old problems, so that everyone feels included in the progress and success of the workplace or clinical area. Inward looking organisations that fail to seek or accept diversity become inflexible and struggle to adjust to change or respond to new situations. Diversity also supports the development of new connections with other professionals, other departments, other institutions, voluntary organisations, clients or their relatives. New approaches to teamwork and wider sets of language skills or interprofessional knowledge may result. Wider professional connections with interprofessional or interdisciplinary relationships foster wider opportunities for clients and patients, greater organisational success and greater cultural awareness as our professional networks are expanded.

WHY DO INTERVIEWS?

Why do we rely upon interviews for staff recruitment? Do they really provide a sound insight into the values and suitability of the employee to the organisation? When we interview a potential employee, we get to hear what they want us to know. Even with the most carefully constructed or structured questions, what we hear at an interview is seldom far from what the potential applicant thinks we want to hear. Is there another or more effective way to find a recruit who will fit well with your organisation?

Another approach is to try and align the employee's values with those of the organisation. This can be achieved by offering values-based scenario events either within the context of the interview or as a separate event beyond or instead of the interview. Here are some staged approaches to this way of applying Congruent Leadership:

- The interviewer(s) could include a question that asks the interviewee if they can describe or list the organisation's values.
- The interviewer(s) could ask a question that explores the interviewee's knowledge of the organisation's values, and asks them to describe how their personal values align or how they see themselves delivering on the values in a work situation.
- The interviewer(s) could ask a question that explores the interviewee's knowledge of the organisation's values, and then asks them to describe how they would respond to a scenario presented to them that tests or explores how they would apply their values to the situation described.
- In this final interview approach, avoid asking if the interviewee knows about the organisation's values and simply present them with a scenario and ask them to describe how they would respond. This will facilitate insight into their values and how they may align or not with the organisation's values, without alerting the interviewee that this is the specific object of the question.

Values-based scenario examples are best designed by the interviewer or interview panel as they will know their own organisation's core values. However, here are two examples that may point to the type of scenario that could be useful:

1. In this organisation, excellent customer service is one of the core values. In this scenario a customer approaches the cash register and attempts to purchase a product with a gift voucher that had expired one week earlier. The customer quickly becomes frustrated when a cashier refuses to accept it. The interviewee is asked to help resolve the issue between the cashier and the customer. How will the potential employee respond?
2. In the second scenario, the value of integrity is tested. A customer gives the casher $50 for a $20 product. The cashier, who is distracted, gives the customer

change from the $50 ($30) and then also gives the original $50 back ($80). The interviewee is the customer. Do they take the bonus or point out the cashier's mistake and return the $50? I would also ask, 'Why?' with whichever response they gave.

The final stage of applying a scenario-based recruitment process is to undertake a small interview to address the main aspects of the process and to check qualifications and general suitability for the position with individual candidates. However, in this approach, a number of candidates are then placed in a 'real-world' scenario whereby they are to role model their response to an ethical or values-based event. This approach will allow candidates to demonstrate their response to the scenario in the context of actually acting upon rather than just talking about their values. This approach allows the employer to put multiple recruits in one place and test out their values by providing an orchestrated and observed event. In addition, the potential employees are tested with other potential employees and their core values will be aligned between and among the group. The employer representatives observe the group as they deal with the scenario and determine the most suitable candidates based on their performance and actions in response to the scenario. The scenario need not be complex, but it will be of more value if it can be as realistic as possible. The scenario may involve actors with set scripts or current employees who can act out their required part. In each case actors or employees in the scenario also provide feedback about the potential employee's 'performance' that will embellish the decision-making capacity of the recruitment team.

This may sound like a lot more work than a standard set of interviews, but the ability to group applicants and place a number of applicants in a scenario situation will potentially streamline the recruitment process. Significantly, it will also mean that new employees will be employed whose values match those of the organisation, saving wasted time with later disciplinary situations or issues of poor or inappropriate performance that are not in keeping with the values of the organisation. Scenario 8.1 is an example of how this could be applied.

SCENARIO 8.1   VALUES-BASED RECRUITMENT

FINDING/ASSESSING CONGRUENT LEADERS

You are recruiting for a ward manager. The core value you are assessing is that your organisation puts families first and has a family-friendly policy that supports its employees when pressing family concerns or family issues arise.

- *Potential employees.* There are six in the group, three male and three female. (All their qualifications and past experiences make them potentially suitable employees although some are more experienced than others.)

(Continued)

(Continued)

- *The scenario.* You are planning an office team-building/teamworking activity to address issues of poor interpersonal communication between staff. The date has been set and resources booked.
- *Scene.* Ward office.
- *Resources.* An actor (female) who is in the early stages of being pregnant and who seems to be at the core of the interpersonal disruption in the ward comes to meet with the group of potential employees to say that she is unable to attend the office team-building event because she has to go for a scan that day. She adds that she is sure she will not need to go to the team-building event because she gets on with everyone 'really well'.
- *Challenge.* How do the six potential recruits deal with the situation? How do they respond to the employee? How do they interact with each other? Do they mention or discuss the values of the organisation and the focus on the organisation being family friendly? Do they discuss their responses or feelings in the presence of the actor, or is she asked to wait outside for a decision? How do the six potential employees demonstrate their emotions and their feelings about this employee or the situation in the ward? Do they all contribute? Are there any that hang back or fail to make their values or views known?

The final stage of the process is to offer feedback to each potential employee about their performance in the scenario, although this is done without giving an indication of the outcome of the interview/recruitment process. It also allows an opportunity to explore why members of the group said or did certain things or responded in the way they did within the scenario.

This approach is not new and it is being used in organisations that recognise that employing anyone because they have the skills or qualifications may be a worse outcome than waiting and finding someone who is a better fit with the organisation's values in the long run. Congruent leaders may not recognise that they are followed because their values are matched by their actions; however, if organisations can search for employees that match their actions with the organisation's values, they will develop a more powerful and successful organisation with a stronger base of employees working to help uphold what the organisation is standing or striving for.

———————— **ACTIVITY 8.2   REFLECTIVE EXERCISE** ————————

Can you think of other approaches to applying Congruent Leadership in practice or in your workplace? Note them down. Apply them.

EXAMPLES OF CONGRUENT LEADERS

John Brown, an American abolitionist who believed in armed insurrection as the most effective way to end the institution of slavery in the United States, may seem like an odd choice to include as an example for a congruent leader and I speculated for some time about the validity and appropriateness of his place in this book. However, he really does fit the mould of a congruent leader even though, as you will see, his methods and tactics may have been faulty.

John Brown was born 9 May 1800 in Connecticut, America. He was raised in Ohio in an area known as the Western Reserve and he learnt early to hunt and trap. He was fond of animals and he lived in a pious community of New Englanders who had come to establish 'godly' settlements in the area. Brown's father worked hard to establish himself and his family and after his mother died when he was eight, Brown looked to his domineering father for support and guidance. Religion and religious fervour featured throughout his life and Brown was fond of reciting scripture. As a young adult Brown was described as being arrogant, having 'self-certitude' and a domineering manner (Horwitz, 2011, p. 13) and while a strict father, his children were said to have 'loved him'.

At the age of 12 he witnessed a slave boy being beaten with iron shovels and this led him to reflect on the wretched, hopeless condition of fatherless and motherless slave children. He also displayed tolerance of America's native inhabitants. However, his views were based less on those of equality and more likely formed early as the product of his father's religious influence. These were based upon Puritan beliefs that established a covenant with God to make America a moral beacon for the world to see and slavery was seen by Calvinist preachers as a threat to their covenant.

John Brown married young and moved his family to a sparsely populated area of Pennsylvania where he and his wife (Dianthe) had six children. John built a home and a shelter for runaway slaves and helped local Native Americans as he built his tannery and raised stock and his family. He was soon established as a leading community figure and civic leader. Sadly, Dianthe died soon after giving birth to their seventh child (who was stillborn) and although John married again less than a year later and had 13 more children with his second wife Mary, his businesses struggled and he was often faced with severe economic hardship. By the 1830s he was distracted and frustrated by economic failings and forces he described as beyond his control, and he began to focus on his determination to help slaves in more significant ways.

He had long viewed slavery as an abomination and unlike his father, who was a pacifist, Brown's beliefs meant that he soon saw that the only solution for the abolition of slavery was an armed insurrection. Brown spent a long time talking about and preaching on the evils of slavery, until in 1856 he had finally become dissatisfied with a pacifist agenda. He said of his fellow abolitionists 'These men are all talk. What we need is action – action!' Provocation was added by the Fugitive Slave Act of 1850 and Brown was provoked to act by leading a small group of volunteers into Kansas during the Bleeding Kansas crisis. There, in response to the attack on the town of Lawrence by pro-slavery forces, Brown and others killed five supporters of slavery at the Potawatomie massacre, before leading anti-slavery groups at the Battle of Black Jack and the Battle of Osawatomie.

During the troubles in Kansas Brown established a strict code of honour for his followers. In it he said (somewhat prophetically) 'Never confess, never betray, never renounce the cause. Stand by one another, and by your friends, while a drop of blood remains: and be hanged, if you must, but tell no tales out of school' (Horwitz, 2011, p. 37).

Brown was a man of conviction. He believed that black people should not be slaves and that the policies of the American government were vacillating on the matter. As such he took matters into his own hands. After the troubles in Kansas, John Brown planned and led a raid on the Federal Armoury at Harpers Ferry on the southern bank of the Potomac River, in Virginia. His plan was to seize the Armoury and distribute weapons to the slaves the group planned to free in the area. The attack had started well, but ultimately failed as Brown's men were killed or captured by pro-slavery townsfolk, the local militia and US Marines led by Robert E. Lee.

Brown and the surviving members of his raiding party were hanged and most historians agree that the raid on Harpers Ferry increased mistrust between the North and South and escalated tension leading up to the American Civil War. Brown was a congruent leader. He was courageous and determined, resolute and persistent. He had his values and beliefs on show and he inspired many others to support and act with him. He was empowered and empathetic and put himself to the fore when action was required. As an abolitionist and devout Christian, he was passionate and energetic and as such he did what he felt were the right things to do. However, the question of his tactics remains one of considerable debate. History books describe him as either a heroic martyr or a madman and terrorist. But he was not a martyr or terrorist, nor mad or insane. He was a passionate man, with a life history that taught him the significance of staying true to his convictions. The key link between John Brown and Congruent Leadership was that he acted, and although his tactics and actions were considered by many to be inappropriate, he at least put his values and beliefs on show through his actions for all to see.

CHAPTER SUMMARY

This chapter has offered some ideas and suggestions for the application of Congruent Leadership in the workplace. It suggests that we should all be clear about what our personal values are, we also need to be clear about and understand the values of the organisation for which we work. Leaders need to role model their values (indeed we all do) and leaders need to be present and visible across a wide spectrum of the workplace for the leader's values to be known. We need to give voice to our values and be sure what we say is consistent (congruent) with what we do and organisations, through their leaders, need to reinforce the organisation's values and behaviours with appropriate rewards. It is also suggested that interviews do not always allow organisations to locate staff with the 'right' values for each organisation and a new approach to interviews (with a focus on testing out potential employees' values) may be required.

SUMMARY: THE
CONGRUENT LEADER

'Too many of our leaders are intellectual street-sweepers – they keep the place nice and tidy, maintaining the status quo and the conventional wisdom, but add nothing to the intellectual and spiritual sum of who we are, what we need and where we're heading as a society. It is the dreamers who are the true leaders.'

Bryce Courtenay, author, *A Recipe for Dreaming* (2007)

INTRODUCTION

Pat Benatar sang in 1983 that 'Love Is a Battlefield'. The workplace may also be a battlefield with clashes over values, objectives, priorities, needs or demands. They need not be, but I have encountered few workplaces where there was not some sort of unrest or even open animosity. The healthcare sector suffers from a range of workplace clashes, perhaps more so than some other fields given the plethora of literature there is about bullying and incivility in the health sector. We have a wide range of different professional disciplines and often significant cost pressures that impact daily on the allocation of scarce resources and valuable time. Health professionals deal with critical life events and ethical and values-based issues daily. Finding and standing by our values may be the only way to truly and safely navigate the minefield that a modern workplace may be.

Healthcare too has a long association with battle, the military and conflict. Nursing has ancient links to the Crusades and the acts of charity by various Orders of Knights. Florence Nightingale became famous as a result of her involvement in the Crimean War. Much of what was learnt about wound care and dealing with trauma comes from conflict or war zones and even the word 'shock' is from a medieval French word that means the point of impact of two large armed groups. Our practice of triage, the development of intensive care units and a host of medications commonly used today have evolved because of healthcare's and health professionals' intersection with the military, conflict and battle. Therefore in this summary chapter I will begin by using some military examples to conclude my discussion of Congruent Leadership.

WATERLOO AND THE SOMME

In Bernard Cornwell's detailed and excellently described book about the Battle of Waterloo *Waterloo: The History of Four Days, Three Armies and Three Battles* (2014) there is a description of the attitude of soldiers towards officers. Often the nineteenth-century British soldier has been described as the scum of the earth, a mindless mass or a whipped underclass that were driven by uncaring and aristocratic officers. Cornwell, though, indicates that this could not have been further from the truth, adding that, while some officers were not respected, most officers came from the middle class and that in many soldiers' letters, diaries and memoirs the soldiers' affection for their officers shines through. Most 'men' and their officers, Cornwell suggests, were on good or respectful terms. Cornwell states that:

> An officer might be wealthy, certainly wealthier that the average private, he was privileged and even, sometimes, aristocratic, yet he still shared the dangers of the battlefield. Officers were expected to lead by example. (Cornwell, 2014, p. 90)

Cornwell adds that some soldiers divided the officers into two classes: the 'come on' and the 'go on', the former being seen as the 'with us' type of leader. One soldier (Rifleman Costello of the 95th Foot Regiment) added that the 'with us' type of leaders were exceedingly rare. While Rifleman Plunket once told an officer, 'The words go on don't benefit a leader sir.' Interestingly, a soldier from the 57th Virginia Regiment in the American Civil War used a similar phrase describing one of their generals with a lacklustre performance and suggesting that they preferred to say, 'Go on boys', but was never heard to say 'Come on, when we were going in to a fight' (Guelzo, 2014, p. 379).

   The words 'go on' don't benefit a leader because they negate the opportunity for the leader to be visible in the heat of battle and to be able to lead by example. Congruent leaders are the 'come on' and 'with us' type of leaders. They are respected because they have their values on display and act on them. As many battlefield officers have discovered, it meant being visible to the 'men' and leading by example. Being seen as a congruent leader means role modelling appropriate professional behaviours and being present in the work or other environments for others to see their values applied in practice.

In the nineteenth century, the British Army seems to have cultivated these types of leader. In John Keegan's wonderful book *The Face of Battle: A Study of Agincourt, Waterloo and the Somme* (1996) he comments on the 'special factors' at play that prompted men of Kitchener's new armies at the Battle of the Somme to leap up and over the parapet. Factors such as the army's cohesion, a sense of mission, a mood of self-sacrifice, local and national patriotism, a degree of self-confidence and credulity were significant. However, Keegan (1996) is clear that paramount in taking the army into battle was the factor of leadership. He describes the type of leadership seen in the First World War, at least in the British Army, as being 'conscious, principled and exemplary' (Keegan, 1996, p. 272). Most of the Kitchener officers came not from the military, but from the extensive British public-school system. They led the way they had learnt. In effect, many were simply being themselves. Keegan (1996) states that:

> ... the first amateur officers provided their untrained soldiers both with an environment and a type of leadership almost identical to those found in a regular, peace time regiment. They organised games for the men, and took part themselves, because that was the public-school recipe for usefully occupying young males in their spare time. They organised competitions between platoons and companies – in cross-country running, rifle shooting, trench digging – because competition was the dynamic of public school life. They saw to the men's food, health, cleanliness, because as seniors they had been taught to do the same for the junior boys. (Keegan, 1996, p. 274)

These officers (leaders) were taking part, being with, being seen, being courageous and leading by example. One description of the Kitchener officers in the First World War was written by Donald Hankey (killed on the Somme in October 1916). He is quoted in Keegan (1996, p. 275–6) as describing the leadership approach of the Kitchener officer as follows:

> He came in the early days ... tall, erect, smiling ... for a few days he just watched. Then he started work. He picked out some of the most awkward ones and ... marched them away by themselves ... His confidence was infectious. He simply could not fail to be understood ... very soon the awkward squad found themselves awkward no longer ... the fact was that he had won his way into our affections. We loved him ... If anyone had a sore foot he would kneel down ... and look at it ... If a blister had to be lanced, he would very likely lance it himself ...'

Here again are some of the attributes of the congruent leader. Hankey describes someone with excellent communication skills, who listened as much as talked, who was approachable, who was visible, who was confident and competent and led by being 'with us', leading with their values and beliefs on show, doing and being seen to do the things that the 'men' respected and required. Clearly Hankey and these officers understood that men could not be 'managed' into battle. It was these types of leaders and this type of leadership that was a crucial factor in prompting the men of Kitchener's armies at the Battle of the Somme to leap up and go 'over the top'.

People in a wide range of occupations and professions, working as they often do at the coalface or in the trenches of their line of work, can likewise not be managed into the more challenging aspects of their work or professional practice. This is not to say management within any work environment is not needed – indeed it is vital. Clearly, all employees need to be managed, but when workers, professionals or employees are dealing with the messy and complex interpersonal and interprofessional spheres of work or practice. It is more effective if interpersonal skills such as being approachable, being seen, being present, being able to communicate clearly and other attributes of Congruent Leadership are applied.

Back at the Battle of Waterloo (fought on 18 June in 1815) it was these factors that helped secure the battle for the allies. Both Von Blücher (the Prussian general) and the Duke of Wellington (the Dutch-British general) offered leadership whereby they were visible, their men saw them and were encouraged by their presence. In addition, Wellington valued order above all else. Order kept the men safe and reduced their risk of being killed or wounded. He demonstrated this at Waterloo by placing his men on the reverse slope of the main ridge when the Dutch-British soldiers were under intense cannon fire. Wellington often fought with smaller armies and he knew the value of protecting the soldiers from wasteful lost of life. His men knew this of him and respected him for his care of their welfare. He also valued the men themselves and as Cornwell states:

> … he valued his men, and they knew that too and many accounts pay tribute to the Duke's presence. When the battle was at its fiercest, when canister and roundshot and musket balls were shredding British-Dutch ranks, then Wellington was frequently just paces away. (2014, p. 217)

However, Napoleon, while present and often visible on the battlefield, left the conduct of the battle to Marshal Nay who wasted his soldiers and cavalry on fruitless and ill-coordinated frontal or peripheral attacks. The battle was a 'close run thing', however, and in the end it was most likely leadership that made the difference and, most significantly, delivered the victory to the allies.

CONGRUENT LEADERSHIP: THE WORKPLACE BATTLE

As suggested above, the office, the classroom, the factory floor, the clinic, the service counter, the ward, or indeed any workplace may not be a war zone and most employees are not in a battle. Or are they? Are references to leadership in Keegan's book, *The Face of Battle* irrelevant when considering leadership in any of these work environments? The situations are vastly different and the circumstances vary considerably. However, the nature of leadership in battle and the nature of leadership while working on a busy medical ward, in a demanding factory production line, a frantic office, a hectic classroom or any workplace could be very similar, which is why the leadership approach for each may be compatible.

Wellington knew that he needed to be present all about the battlefield to fortify and bolster his troops' courage and resilience. British officers on the Somme knew that they needed to be the ones to care for the 'men' and to share their rations, the suffering, the cold, the privation and their fate. In both cases this created a sense of being in the 'fight' together. It created a unified and common purpose and a together-ness that was linked by their values and beliefs that grew from understanding what they were fighting for and from a mutual respect of the risks each other were taking.

The First World War created another kind of general. They were known as the château generals and they were known as such because they never (or rarely) came to the battlefield. They made their plans and conducted the war out of artillery range and in comparative safety and comfort in the numerous French châteaux, often well to the rear of the fighting.

Managers can also be leaders. However, when managers are found mainly in their offices, removed from the shopfloor, factory bench, hospital ward, classroom chaos and front-line operations of an organisation they may sometimes be compared to the château generals. They are vital for the business to function and for the organisation to run, but do they employ a different leadership approach? The theory of Congruent Leadership may be harder to apply to their leadership style or requirements. They employ other approaches to leadership; transactional, transformational and situational leadership. These are valid and appropriate leadership theories, but they seem less well suited to the types of leadership seen or required by employees and workers in the office, the classroom, the factory floor, the service counter, the hospital ward, at the coalface or in the trenches of the modern workplace. The key to this issue is that if the leader's values differ from those of the employees, tension and dissatisfaction will result.

Scenario 9.1 is an example of a senior health service manager who was able to apply Congruent Leadership and remain effective. Indeed she achieved great success, because she led with her values and beliefs on show and held them evident in the delivery of her leadership role.

SCENARIO 9.1   A CONGRUENT LEADER AND A HEALTH SERVICE MANAGER

The Chief Nurse and Midwife (CN&M) in Western Australia between 2009 and 2014 was in my view a congruent leader. She was very well liked and made a point of getting to know nurses and midwives at all levels. She was not seen as aloof or remote from the real world of clinical practice. She undertook to improve patient care in Western Australia by encompassing the collective insight and participation of nurses and midwives across the state. She really was a 'clinician's chief nurse'. She

(Continued)

(Continued)

demonstrated Congruent Leadership. It was evident in her actions that she was capable, compassionate and dedicated and that she had the best interests of patients and nurses as a core value. The CN&M was down to earth in her approach to fellow nurses and midwives and very approachable. She could mix with nurses or midwives as well as key politicians and I never once felt she was being false or disingenuous. She valued what nurses and midwives could contribute to the welfare of Western Australians and she acted on her values to demonstrate leadership that was consistent with her beliefs and focused on the contribution that nurses and midwives could make to the direction and welfare of the Health Service in Western Australia.

When teachers care about the needs of the children they teach, and managers (head teachers) seem not to recognise the teacher's pleas for additional resources to meet the children's needs, this can cause a clash of values. When a factory worker is asked to undertake repeated overtime that restricts the worker's time with his family and means that when the worker is with his family he is tired and stressed, this can result in a clash of values. When a manager is under pressure to cut the budget and the impact of this is that services and time with clients is cut, this can result in a clash of values. When ward staff are off sick and a manager asks a nurse with a full patient load to cover staffing issues on another ward, this can lead to a clash of values. More than vision, a person is driven to do what they do because they hold convictions, values or beliefs that govern how they see the world (their workplace, their home, their community) and their place within it. Recognising that leaders who are able to demonstrate a stance in relation to their values and beliefs are commonly followed because they put these into action. This places a priority on understanding Congruent Leadership as a primary objective for any organisation, industry, business, institution or person who wishes to lead well.

CLOSING THE LOOP

The theory of Congruent Leadership developed from the results of a number of research studies (outlined in Chapter 2) that have explored leadership from the perspective of a number of various health professional disciplines. The initial research was undertaken with registered nurses at a large acute hospital in the UK between 2001 and 2004. This was followed by five further research projects that explored the phenomenon of clinical leadership from the perspective of paramedics (in 2008), senior registered nurses and managers in the aged care arena (in 2012), ambulance volunteers (in 2013) and allied health professionals, mainly dietetics, occupational therapists, physiotherapists, social workers, podiatrists and speech therapists (between 2014 and 2015), in Australia and rural and remote nurses in Western NSW (Australia) in 2017. It was soon clear that none of the previously established leadership theories described or supported the results that began to emerge from the research. As such, a new leadership theory focused on values-based leadership was needed.

At the time I started to explore leadership that was not related to management or tied to positions of authority, the dominant leadership theory supporting healthcare leadership was transformational leadership. However, as discussed in Chapter 4, transformational leadership theory is based on the leader's vision and how their vision is communicated to those who see them as leaders (or are told they are their leaders, e.g. managers). In the course of the leadership research undertaken and presented in support of Congruent Leadership theory, having a vision or being visionary was seldom identified by respondents as being relevant or significant. Instead, the leaders I encountered (shopfloor, coalface or bedside leaders) were rarely described as having or requiring the attribute of being visionary. This led to the conclusion that established leadership theories that rested on 'vision' as the basis for leadership theory were unable to describe the type of leadership displayed by this type of leader (or any leaders, at any level, without authority, power, a big office or a large badge).

FINAL WORDS

The research indicated that clinically focused nurses and a range of health professionals who stand decisively and clearly on the foundations of their values and beliefs can be seen to be expressing Congruent Leadership. They may have simply stood by their values, working – not because they wanted to change the world but because they knew that what they were doing was the right thing and their actions were making a difference. When acting out or role modelling their values and beliefs (even subconsciously) something was happening in their relationships with their clients, patients or colleagues that gave a clear signal about what they believed or what their values were. This links Congruent Leadership with the expression of emotional intelligence and values-based relationship building.

Congruent leaders stand by their values and this is clear in the execution of their actions. They put their hands where their heart is, walk their walk and act out and follow through with what they believe to be right. These leaders are not selling a vision or communicating a path for others to follow, they are living their vision and walking the path themselves, role modelling with commitment, conviction and determination what they believe is the right thing to do. They are congruent leaders.

EXAMPLES OF CONGRUENT LEADERS

There are many others I could have cited as examples of congruent leaders. You might like to explore their lives and examples of their leadership after reading this book. I could have discussed Mahatma Gandhi (Indian political and spiritual leader), Harriet Beecher-Stowe (author of *Uncle Tom's Cabin*), Dr Martin Luther King (American civil rights leader), Galileo Galilei (scientist and reformer), Harriet Tubman (a civil rights activist during the American Civil War, and women's sufferage fighter), Edith Cavell (a nun who was murdered by German forces in the First World War), Mary Wollstonecraft (English writer, philosopher and advocate of women's rights), George Washington (American statesman and soldier who served as the first President of the United States from 1789 to 1797 and was one of the Founding Fathers of the United States), Albert-Marie Edmond Guèrisse, also known as 'Patrick O'Leary' (leader of a 'freedom line' out of Nazi occupied Europe during the Second World War), Emmeline Pankhurst (suffragette and women's rights activist), Dian Fossey and Jane Goodall (prominent researchers on and advocates for primates), Dorethea Dix (American activist on behalf of the indigent mentally ill), Chai Jing (Chinese journalist, host, author and environmental activist), Franklin D. Roosevelt (American statesman and political leader), John Simpson Kirkpatrick (a stretcher bearer with the 1st Australian Division during the Gallipoli Campaign in the First World War), Helen Keller (American author, political activist and lecturer who was the first deaf-blind person to earn a bachelor of arts degree), Agnes Humbert, Jean Cassou, Jean Cabut and Stephan Charbonnier (members of the French Resistance during the Second World War), Emily Murphy (Canadian women's rights activist, jurist and author), Oskar Schindler (German industrialist and a member of the Nazi Party who is credited with saving the lives of 1,200 Jews during the Holocaust).

The reality is that there are thousands of people who are congruent leaders. They may not all be front-line, coalface, action-focused leaders, but they all make a difference to ordinary people by caring more than they think is wise, risking more than they think is safe, knowing more than is reasonably required, dreaming more than others think is practical, and giving more of themselves than might be considered prudent. These are congruent leaders. They are not 'gunnas', as in they are not people who are (going to do something) or in Australian parlance, 'gunna' do something. They are people who do it. They are doers! They do not depend on titles, big offices or high-paid administrative or management positions. However, in my experience, few of these things are a prerequisite for the application of excellent leadership or as a tool for congruent leaders to lead well.

I would like to include one final example of a congruent leader. In keeping with the military tone of this chapter the person I would like to discuss is Lieutenant Colonel Lucy Giles. She is the first female commander of the famous British military training college Sandhurst. Lt Col. Giles explained her approach to training future officers in the British army as 'train in, rather than select out'. Reed (2018, p. 131) explains: 'The approach is about spotting the potential in people and giving them the opportunities to develop, rather than looking for people who are the finished article and getting rid of the rest.' 'Fundamentally,' Lt Col. Giles explains, 'everything comes down to values. The army has a set – courage, discipline, respect for others, integrity, loyalty and selfless commitment.' Her job is to make sure these are ingrained. According to Reed (2018, p. 132) she describes her leadership approach as, 'drink more tea', i.e. getting out from behind her desk and spending time with the troops, to have a brew and a chat, to find out what is going on with them, be alongside them, both literally and figuratively, in the trenches. She indicates that having values and living up to them and helping others do the same is what makes a great solider (nurse, health professional, sales assistant, manager, firefighter, paramedic, etc.). Reed offers this quote from Lt Col. Giles:

> Life for me is about doing the right thing, on a difficult day, when no one is looking. If you do something or walk by something that you know is not right, then you're ultimately cheating and undermining your own self. If you do the right thing, no matter what the outcome, your confidence always grows. And you have a better life that way. So just make sure you are always honest with yourself. And make sure you always do the right thing. (Reed, 2018, p. 132).

CHAPTER SUMMARY

Congruent Leadership offers a genuine leadership solution for modern healthcare and other workplaces and political arenas. It bases the leader's influence upon their values, is connected to their emotions and is demonstrated by their actions. In a very real way Congruent Leadership allows or encourages leaders to focus on their values and, in the process, build a workplace, community or society that will facilitate their followers to leave the world in a better place. Congruent leaders do not set out to change the world, but to be better people in the world, and as a result the world is generally better off for the mark they make while following their values.

Unfortunately, it may be easy to diminish the importance of values and beliefs in the glare of government reform, competing political agendas, financial constraints, workplace financial targets or cuts, technological advances, artificial intelligence and other practical or imagined constraints. However, these are the very obstacles leaders really need to get to grips with if solutions to the modern workplace or political environment are to be found. Congruent leaders are out there, they are always there, in the shadows, in the wings, by the bedside, at the service counter, in the classroom, in the boardroom, in the clinic, on the factory floor, in the office. This book hopes to illuminate their presence and identify them so that we can recognise them and understand their place as leaders, even without the title, big office or authority.

They have their values on show, they are committed, passionate, persistent, dynamic, empowered, energetic, approachable, charismatic, inspirational and motivational. They do the right thing. They are visible and role model the values they hold dear. They are effective communicators, listening well and remaining calm in times of crisis. They know the important parts of their work role and they can do them well. They can make key decisions when needed and while they may not intend to change work practices, their main contribution is to role model their values with conviction and dedication, so that others recognise and can follow their values and beliefs as a shining light for others to follow.

That said, things often do change when congruent leaders make a stand. As with Tank Man or Rosa Parks, it is not always their intention to make a change so much as to make a stand. Rosa Parks said she wasn't angry, she just felt determined to take an opportunity to let it be known that she didn't want to be treated this way anymore, and she had no idea how people would react to her arrest. What Rosa didn't know was that she was a leader and that she had followers. Congruent leaders often don't know this either. In my initial research, only half of the leaders who were identified as such recognised themselves as leaders. I suspect the people who arrested Rosa Parks didn't know they were dealing with a leader either. In the same way, I wonder if managers, educators, organisations, HR departments, CEOs or department heads recognise the leaders who are in their workplaces, influencing and leading their colleagues or workmates with their own values and shaping the organisation's culture.

However, I feel it is vital that managers, educators, organisations, HR departments, CEOs or department heads (and the congruent leaders themselves) recognise the virtual army of people in the workforce who are leading because they match their values with their actions. Congruent leaders are out there driving, developing and supporting innovation and change and making a difference in all workplaces and walks of life. Organisational goals and innovation can best be led by congruent leaders who are recognised and valued for the contribution they bring, or can bring, to an organisation at every level, not just as facilitators of the work they are employed to do.

The examples throughout this book are offered to clarify Congruent Leadership and how clinical leaders can be seen as effective and vital leaders, in any business, organisation, workplace, institution or industry and who can be found at any level, in any position and in any area because they lead, by putting their values on show, so that others see the connection between their values and the things they do.

REFERENCES

CHAPTER 1

Adair, J. (1998) *Effective Leadership*. London: Pan Books.

Adair, J. (2002a) *Inspirational Leadership*. London: Thorogood Books.

Adair, J. (2002b) *Effective Strategic Leadership: An Essential Path to Success Guided by the World's Greatest Leaders*. London: Pan Books.

Allan, J. (1992) 'Fordism and modern industry', in J. Allan, P. Abraham and P. Lewis (eds), *Political and Economic Forms of Modernity*. Cambridge: Polity Press.

American Association of Critical-Care Nurses (2005) 'AACN standards for establishing and sustaining healthy work environments: a journey to excellence', *American Journal of Critical Care*, 14 (3): 187–97. Available online at: http://ajcc.aacnjournals.org/content/14/3/187. short

Anderson, R.J. (2003) 'Building hospital–physician relationships through servant leadership', *Frontiers of Health Service Management*, 20 (2): 43.

Avolio, B.J. and Gardener, W.L. (2005) 'Authentic leadership development: getting to the root of positive forms of leadership', *Leadership Quarterly*, 16 (3): 315–38.

Banks, H. (1982) *The Rise and Fall of Freddie Laker*. London: Faber & Faber.

Bass, B.M. (1985) *Leadership and Performance Beyond Expectations*. New York: Free Press.

Bass, B.M. (1990) 'From transactional to transformational leadership: learning to share the vision', *Organisational Dynamics*, 18: 19–31.

Bell, D. and Ritchie, R. (1999) *Towards Effective Subject Leadership in Primary School*. Buckingham: Open University Press.

Bennis, W. and Nanus, B. (1985) *Leaders: The Strategies for Taking Charge*. New York: Harper & Row.

Bennis, W., Parikh, J. and Lessem, R. (1995) *Beyond Leadership: Balancing Economics, Ethics and Ecology*. Oxford: Blackwell Business.

Bernhard, L.A. and Walsh M. (1990) *Leadership: The Key to the Professionalization of Nursing*. London: Mosby.

Bhindi, N. and Duignan, P. (1997) 'Leadership for a new century: authenticity, intentionality, spirituality and sensibility', *Educational Management and Administration*, 25 (4): 117–32.

Blake, R.R. and McCanse A.A. (1991) *Leadership Dilemmas – Grid Solutions*. Houston, TX: Gulf Publishing.

Blake, R.R. and Mouton, J.S. (1964) The Managerial Grid, Houston, TX: Gulf Publishing, in P.G. Northouse (2016) *Leadership: Theory and Practice*, 7th edn. London: Sage.

Blanchard, K., Zigarmi, P. and Zigarmi, D. (1994), *Leadership and the One-minute Manager*. London: HarperCollins Business.

Branson, R. (1998) *Losing My Virginity*. London: Virgin.

Burns, J.M. (1978) *Leadership*. New York: Harper & Row.

Campbell, P.T. and Rudisill, P.T. (2005) 'Servant leadership: a critical component for nurse leaders', *Nurse Leader, 3* (3): 27–9.

Cantwell, J. (2015) *Leadership in Action*. Carlton, Vic.: Melbourne University Press.

Carson, C. (ed.) (1999) *The Autobiography of Martin Luther King Junior*. London: Little, Brown.

Carwardine, R.J. (2003) *Lincoln – Profiles in Power*. Harlow: Pearson Longman.

Casida, J. and Parker, J. (2011) 'Staff nurse perceptions of nurse manager leadership styles and outcomes', *Journal of Nursing Management, 19*: 478–86.

Clemmer, J. and McNeil, A. (1989) *Leadership Skills for Every Manager*. London: Piatkus Books.

Covey, S.R. (1992) *Principle-centred Leadership*. London: Simon & Schuster.

Danzig, R.J. (2000) *The Leader Within You*. Hollywood, FL: Lifetime Books Frederick Fell.

Day, C., Harris, A., Hadfield, M., Tolley, H. and Beresford, J. (2000) *Leading Schools in Times of Change*. Buckingham: Open University Press.

D'Este, C. (1996) *A Genius for War: A Life of General George S. Patton*. London: HarperCollins.

Downton, J.V. (1973) *Rebel Leadership: Commitment and Charisma in a Revolutionary Process*. New York: Free Press.

Dublin, R. (1968) *Human Relations in Administration*, 2nd edn. Englewood Cliffs, NJ: Prentice-Hall.

Duke, D.L. (1986) 'The aesthetics of leadership', *Educational Administration Quarterly, 22* (1): 7 – 27.

Eicher-Catt, D. (2005) 'The myth of servant leadership: a feminist perspective', *Women and Language, 28* (1): 17–26.

Fest, J. (1974) *Hitler*. London: Weidenfeld & Nicolson.

Fiedler, F.E. (1967) *A Theory of Leadership Effectiveness*. New York: McGraw-Hill.

Freshwater, D., Graham, I. and Esterhuizen, P. (2009) 'Educating leaders for global health care', in V. Bishop (ed.) *Leadership for Nursing and Allied Health Care Professions*. Berkshire: Open University Press/McGraw-Hill Education.

Fuda, P. (2014) Leadership Transformed: *How Ordinary Managers Become Extraordinary Leaders*. London: Profile Books.

Gallagher, G.W., Engle, S.D., Krick, R.K. and Glatthaar, J.T. (2003) *The American Civil War: This Mighty Scourge of War*. Oxford: Osprey.

Galton, F. (1869) Hereditary Genius, 1st edn. New York: Appleton, in M. Morrison (1993), *Professional Skills for Leadership: Foundations for a Successful Career*. St Louis, LA: Mosby.

Geneen, H. & Moscow, A. (1984) *Managing*. Doubleday. New York.

George, B. (2003) *Authentic Leadership: Rediscovering the Secrets to Creating Lasting Value*. San Francisco: Jossey-Bass.

Goertz Koerner, J. (2010) 'Reflections on transformational leadership', *Journal of Holistic Nursing, 28* (1): 68.

Goleman, D. (1996) *Emotional Intelligence*. New York: Bloomsbury Press.

Goleman, D., Boyatzis, R. and McKee, A. (2002) *The New Leaders*. London: Time Warner Paperback.

Gonzalez, M. (2012) *Mindful Leadership*. Ontario: John Wiley & Sons Canada.

Grabsky, P. (1993) *The Great Commanders*. London: Boxtree.

Greenfield, T.B. (1986) 'Leaders and school: wilfulness and non-natural order in organizations', in T.J. Sergiovanni and J. E. Corbally (eds), *Leadership and Organizational Culture: New Perspectives on Administration Theory and Practice*. Chicago: University of Chicago Press.

Greenleaf, R.K. (1977) *Servant Leadership: A Journey into the Nature of Legitimate Power and Greatness*. Mahwah, NJ: Paulist Press.

Grint, K. (2000) *The Arts of Leadership*. Oxford: Oxford University Press.

Grossman, S. and Valiga, T.M. (2013) *The New Leadership Challenge: Creating the Future of Nursing*, 4th edn. Philadephia, PA: FA Davis.

Handy, C. (1999) *Understanding Organisations*, 3rd edn. London: Penguin Books.

Hanse, J.J., Harlin, U., Jarebratnt, C., Ulin, K. and Winkel, J. (2015) 'The impact of servant leadership dimensions on leader–member exchange among health care professionals', *Journal of Nursing Management*. Accessed April 2016. doi: 10.1111/jonm.12304.

Harvey, A.D. (1998) 'Napoleon – the myth', *History Today*, 48 (1): 27–32.

Hersey, P. and Blanchard, K. (1982) *Management of Organisational Behaviour*. Englewood Cliffs, NJ: Prentice-Hall.

Hibbert, C. (1998) *Nelson – A Personal History*. London: Penguin.

House, R.J. (1976) A Theory of Charismatic Leadership, in J.G. Hunt, A. Kakabadse and N. Kakabadse (1999), *Essence of Leadership*. London: International Thomson Business Press.

House, R.J. and Mitchell, T.R. (1974) 'Path–goal theory of leadership', *Journal of Contemporary Business*, Autumn, pp. 81–97.

Hutchinson, M. and Jackson, D. (2012) 'Transformational leadership in nursing: towards a more critical interpretation', *Nursing Inquiry*, 20 (1): 11–22.

Jones, L. and Bennet, C.L. (2012) *Leadership in Health and Social Care: An Introduction for Emerging Leaders*. Banbury: Lantern Publishers.

Kakabadse, A. and Kakabadse, N. (1999) *Essence of Leadership*. London: International Thomson Business Press.

Kerfoot, K. (2004) 'The shelf life of leaders', *Medical Surgical Nursing*, 13 (5): 348–51.

Kirkpatrick, S.A. and Locke, E.A. (1991) 'Leadership: do traits really matter?', *Academy of Management Executive*, 5: 48–60.

Kotter, J.P. (1990) 'What leaders really do', *Harvard Business Review on Leadership*. Boston, MA: Harvard Business School Press, pp. 37–60.

Kouzes, J.M. and Posner, B.Z. (2003) *The Leadership Challenge*, 3rd edn. San Francisco: Jossey-Bass.

Krause, D.G. (2000) *The Way of the Leader*. London: Nicholas Brealey.

Lacey, R. (1986) *Ford*. London: Heinemann.

Lavoie-Tremblay, M., Fernet, C., Lavigne, G.L. and Austin, S. (2015) 'Transformational and abusing leadership practices: impacts on novice nurses, quality of care and intention to leave', *Journal of Advanced Nursing*, 73 (3): 582–92.

Leigh, A. and Maynard, M. (1995) *Leading Your Team: How to Involve and Inspire Teams*. London: Nicholas Brealey.

Lett, M. (2002) 'The concept of clinical leadership', *Contemporary Nurse*, 12 (1): 6–20.

Lewin, K. (1948) *Resolving Social Conflicts: Selected Papers on Group Dynamics*, ed. G.W. Lewin. New York: Harper & Row.

Lipman, J. (1964) 'Leadership administration', in E.E. Griffiths (ed.), *Behavioral Science and Educational Administration*. Chicago: University of Chicago Press.

Mandela, N. (1994) *Long Walk to Freedom*. London: Little, Brown.

Man, J. (2010) *The Leadership Secrets of Genghis Khan*. London: Bantam Books.

Mann, R.D. (1959) 'A review of the relationship between personality and performance in small groups', *Psychological Bulletin*, 56: 402–10.

Marshall, E. (2011) *Leadership in Nursing: From Expert Clinician to Influential Leader*. New York: Springer.

Maxwell, J. (2002) *The 21 Irrefutable Laws of Leadership Workbook*. Nashville: TN: Thomas Nelson.

Morgan, G. (1986) *Images of Organizations*. Beverly Hills, CA: Sage.

National Health Service Confederation (1999) Consultation: The Modern Values of Leadership and Management in the NHS. London: NHS Confederation and the Nuffield Trust.

Northouse, P.G. (2016) *Leadership: Theory and Practice*, 7th edn. London: Sage.

Pedler, M., Burgoyne, J. and Boydell, T. (2004) *A Manager's Guide to Leadership*. Berkshire: McGraw-Hill Professional.

Peete, D. (2005) 'Needed: servant leaders', *Nursing Homes*, 54 (7): 8–10.

Pondy, L.R. (1978) 'Leadership is a language game', in M.W. McCall Jr and M.M. Lombardo (eds), *Leadership: Where Else Can We Go?* Durham, NC: Duke University Press.

Rafferty, A.M. (1993) Leading Questions: A Discussion Paper on the Issues of Nurse Leadership. London: Kings Fund Centre.

Rigolosi, E. (2013) *Management and Leadership in Nursing and Health Care: An Experimental Approach*, 3rd edn. New York: Springer.

Robinson, C.A. (2006) 'The leader within', *Journal of Trauma Nursing*, 13 (1): 35–7.

Ross, E.J., Fitzpatrick, J.J., Click, E.R., Krouse, H.J. and Clavelle, J.T. (2014) 'Transformational leadership practices of nurse leaders in professional nursing associations', *Journal of Nursing Administration*, 44 (4): 201–6.

Sarros, J. and Butchatsky, O. (1996) *Leadership: Australia's Top CEOs Finding Out What Makes Them the Best*. Pymble, NSW: Harper Business.

Shirley, M.R. (2006) 'Authentic leaders creating healthy work environments for nursing practice', *American Journal of Critical Care*, 15 (3): 256–68.

Smith, D. (1999) 'Leadership is a hard act to follow', *Sunday Times*, 'News Review', 18 July, p. 6.

Sofarelli, D. and Brown, D. (1998) 'The need for nursing leadership in uncertain times', *Journal of Nursing Management*, 6: 201–7.

Spears, L.C. (ed.) (1995) *Reflections on Leadership: How Robert Greenleaf's Theory of Servant Leadership Influenced Today's Top Management Thinkers*. New York: John Wiley & Sons.

Stanley, D. (2006) 'Recognising and defining clinical nurse leaders', *British Journal of Nursing*, 15 (2): 108–11.

Stanley, D. (2011) *Clinical Leadership: Innovation into Action*. South Yarra: Palgrave Macmillan.

Stanley, D. (2017) *Clinical Leadership in Nursing and Healthcare*. Oxford: Wiley Blackwell.

Stanton, E., Lemer, C. and Mountford, J. (2010) *Clinical Leadership: Bridging the Divide*. London: Quay Books.

Stogdill, R.M. (1948) 'Personal factors associated with leadership: a survey of the literature', *Journal of Psychology*, 25: 35–71.

Stogdill, R.M. (1950) Leadership, Membership and Organisation, Psychological Bulletin No. 47, in M. Crawford, L. Kydd and C. Riches, *Leadership and Teams in Educational Management*. Buckingham: Open University Press.

Stogdill, R.M. (1974) Handbook of Leadership. New York: Free Press, in M. Crawford, L. Kydd and C. Riches, *Leadership and Teams in Educational Management*. Buckingham: Open University Press.

Swanwick, T. and McKimm, J. (2011) *ABC of Clinical Leadership*. Oxford: Wiley-Blackwell.

Swearingen, S. and Liberman, A. (2004) 'Nursing leadership: serving those who serve others', *Health Care Manager*, 23 (2): 100.

Tannenbaum, R. and Schmidt, W.H. (1958) 'How to choose a leadership pattern', *Harvard Business Review*, 36: 95–101.

Tayeb, M.H. (1996) *The Management of a Multicultural Workforce*. Chichester: Wiley.

Thorne, M. (2006) 'What kind of leader are you?', *Topics in Emergency Medicine*, 28 (2): 104–10.

Thyer, G. (2003) 'Dare to be different: transformational leadership may hold the key to reducing the nursing shortage', *Journal of Nursing Management*, 11: 73–9.

Tinkham, M.R. (2013) 'The road to magnet: encouraging transformational leadership', *ACRN Journal*, 98 (2): 186–8.

Useem, M. (1998) *The Leadership Moment*. Toronto: Times Business Books/Random House.

Vroom, V.H. and Yetton, P. (1973) *Leadership and Decision Making*. Pittsburgh, PA: University of Pittsburgh Press.

Walker, T. (2006) 'Servant leaders', *Managed Healthcare Executive*, 16 (3): 20–6.

Weberg, D. (2010) 'Transformational leadership and staff retention: an evidence review with implications for healthcare systems', *Nursing Administration Quarterly*, 34 (3): 246.

Wedderburn-Tate, C. (1999) *Leadership in Nursing*. London: Churchill Livingstone.

Welford, C. (2002) 'Matching theory to practice', *Nursing Management*, 9 (4): 7–11.

Weng, R.-H., Huang, C.-Y., Chen, L.-M. and Chang, L.-Y. (2015) 'Exploring the impact of transformational leadership on nurse innovation behaviour: a cross-sectional study', *Journal of Nursing Management*, 23: 427–39.

Wong, C. and Cummings, G. (2009) 'Authentic leadership: a new theory for nursing or back to basics?', *Journal of Health Organisations and Management*, 23 (50): 522.

Yoder-Wise, P.S. (2015) *Leading and Management in Nursing*, 6th edn. St Louis, LA: Mosby.

Zaleznik, A. (1977) 'Managers and leaders: are they different?', *Harvard Business Review on Leadership*. Boston: Harvard Business School Press, pp. 61–88.

CHAPTER 2

Bhindi, N. and Duignan, P. (1997) 'Leadership for a new century: authenticity, intentionality, spirituality and sensibility', *Educational Management and Administration*, 25 (4): 117–32.

George, B. (2003) *Authentic Leadership: Rediscovering the Secrets to Creating Lasting Value*. San Francisco: Jossey-Bass.

Kouzes, J.M. and Posner, B.Z. (2010) *The Truth About Leadership: The No-fads, Heart of the Matter Facts You Need to Know*. San Francisco: Jossey-Bass.

Mahoney, J. (2001) 'Leadership skills for the 21st century', *Journal of Nursing Management*, 9: 269–71.

Marriner-Tomey, A. (2009) *Guide to Nursing Management and Leadership*, 8th edn. St Louis, MO Mosby: Elsevier.

National Health Service National Patient Safety Agency (2004) *Seven Steps to Patient Safety: A Guide for NHS Staff*. London: HM Stationery Office.

O'Reilly, C. and Pfeffer, J. (2000) *Hidden Power*. Harvard: Harvard Business School Press.

Pondy, L.R. (1978) 'Leadership is a language game', in M.W. McCall Jr and M.M. Lombardo (eds), *Leadership: Where Else Can We Go?* Durham, NC: Duke University Press.

Rich, V.L. (2008) Chapter 20c: 'Creation of a patient safety culture: a nurse executive leadership imperative'. Available at: www.ahrq.gov/qual/nurseshdbk/doc/rich_vcpsc.pdh

Stanley, D. (2006a) 'In command of care: clinical nurse leadership explored', *Journal of Research in Nursing*, 2 (1): 20–39.

Stanley, D. (2006b) 'In command of care: towards the theory of congruent leadership', *Journal of Research in Nursing*, 11 (2): 134–44.

Stanley, D. (2008) 'Congruent leadership: values in action', *Journal of Nursing Management*, 16: 519–24.

Stanley, D. (2011) *Clinical Leadership: Innovation into Action*. Melbourne: Palgrave Macmillan.

Stanley, D. (2017) *Clinical Leadership in Nursing and Healthcare: Values into Action.* Oxford: Wiley Blackwell.

Stanton, E., Lemer, C. and Mountford, J. (2010) *Clinical Leadership: Bridging the Divide.* London: Quay Books.

Victorian Quality Council (2005) Developing the Clinical Leader's Role in Clinical Governance: A Guide for Clinicians and Health Services. Victorian Department of Health.

CHAPTER 3

Cantwell, J. (2015) *Leadership in Action.* Carlton, Vic.: Melbourne University Press.

Distinti, M. (2011) *Leadership Lessons of Abraham Lincoln.* New York: Skyhorse Publishing.

Goleman, D., Boyatzis, R. and McKee, A. (2013) *Primal Leadership: Unleashing the Power of Emotional Intelligence.* Boston, MA: Harvard Business School Press.

Guelzo, A.C. (2014) *Gettysburg: The Last Invasion.* New York: First Vintage Books Edition.

Rafferty, A.M. (1993) Leading Questions: A Discussion Paper on the Issues of Nurse Leadership. London: Kings Fund Centre.

CHAPTER 4

Antrobus, S. and Kitson, A. (1999) 'Nursing leadership: influencing and shaping health policy and nursing practice', *Journal of Advanced Nursing,* 29 (3): 746–53.

Bass, B.M. (1985) *Leadership and Performance Beyond Expectations.* New York: Free Press.

Bass, B.M. (1990) 'From transactional to transformational leadership: learning to share the vision', *Organisational Dynamics,* 18: 19–31.

Bennis, W. and Nanus, B. (1985) *Leaders: The Strategies for Taking Charge.* New York: Harper & Row.

Berlin, I. (1953) *The Hedgehog and the Fox.* London: Weidenfeld & Nicolson.

Bhindi, N. and Duignan, P. (1997) 'Leadership for a new century: authenticity, intentionality, spirituality and sensibility', *Educational Management and Administration,* 25 (4): 117–32.

Burns, J.M. (1978) *Leadership.* New York: Harper & Row.

Cantwell, J. (2015) *Leadership in Action.* Carlton, Vic.: Melbourne University Press.

Clark. L. (2008) 'Clinical leadership, values, beliefs and vision', *Nursing Management,* 15 (7): 30–5.

Day, C., Harris, A., Hadfield, M., Tolley, H. and Beresford, F.L. (2000) *Leading Schools in Times of Change.* Buckingham: Open University Press.

Department of Health (2013) The NHS Constitution for England. Available from: https://www.gov.uk/government/publications/the-nhs-constitution-for-england/the-nhsconstitution-for-england (Accessed 31st March 2017)

Downton, J.V. (1973) *Rebel Leadership: Commitment and Charisma in a Revolutionary Process.* New York: Free Press.

Frankel, A. (2008) 'What leadership styles should senior nurses develop?', *Nursing Times,* 104 (35): 23–4.

Gentile, M.C. (2010) *Giving Voice to Values: How to Speak Your Mind When You Know What's Right.* New Haven, CT: Yale University Press.

George, B. (2003) *Authentic Leadership – Rediscovering the Secrets to Creating Lasting Value.* San Francisco: Jossey-Bass.

Hall, M.L. (2005) 'Shaping organisational culture: a practitioner's perspective', *Peak Development Consulting,* 2 (1): 1–16.

House, R.J. (1976) 'A theory of charismatic leadership', in J.G. Hunt, A. Kakabadse and N. Kakabadse (eds), *Essence of Leadership*. London: International Thomson Business Press.

Kouzes, J.M. and Posner, B.Z. (2010) *The Truth About Leadership: The No-fads, Heart of the Matter Facts You Need to Know*. San Francisco: Jossey-Bass.

NHS England/Nursing Directorate (2013) Compassion in Practice – One year On. Available from: www.england.nhs.uk/wp-content/uploads/2016/05/cip-one-year-on.pdf (accessed August 2017).

Northhouse, P. G. (2016) *Leadership Theory and Practice*, 7th edn. London: Sage.

O'Reilly, C. and Pfeffer, J. (2000) *Hidden Power*. Cambridge, MA: Harvard Business School Press.

Pendleton, D. and King, J. (2002) 'Values and leadership: education and debate', *British Medical Journal*, 325: 1352–5.

Sarros, J. and Butchatsky, O. (1996) *Leadership: Australia's Top CEOs Finding Out What Makes Them the Best*. Pymble, NSW: Harper Business.

Stanley, D. (2004) 'Clinical leadership: a pilot study explored', *Paediatric Nursing*, 16 (3): 39–42.

Stanley, D. (2006a) 'In command of care: clinical nurse leadership explored', *Journal of Research in Nursing*, 2 (1): 20–39.

Stanley, D. (2006b) In command of care: towards the theory of congruent leadership', *Journal of Research in Nursing*, 11 (2): 134–44.

Stanley, D. (2008) 'Congruent leadership: values in action', *Journal of Nursing Management*, 16: 519–24.

Stanley, D. (2011) *Clinical Leadership: Innovation into Action*. Melbourne: Palgrave Macmillan.

Stanley, D. (2017) *Clinical Leadership in Nursing and Healthcare: Values into Action*. Oxford: Wiley Blackwell.

Vaismoradi, M., Griffiths, P., Turunen, H. and Jordan, S. (2016) 'Transformational leadership in nursing and medication safety education: a discussion paper', *Journal of Nursing Management*, 24: 970–80.

CHAPTER 5

Bhindi, N. and Duignan, P. (1997) 'Leadership for a new century: authenticity, intentionality, spirituality and sensibility', *Educational Management and Administration*, 25 (4): 117–32.

Bishop, V. (ed.) (2009a) *Leadership in Nursing and Allied Health Care Professions*. Open University Press, Chapter 2: 'Leadership and management: a new mutiny?'. Maidenhead, Berkshire.

Bishop, V. (ed.) (2009b) *Leadership in Nursing and Allied Health Care Professions*. Open University Press, Chapter 7: 'Clinical leadership and the theory of congruent leadership'. Maidenhead, Berkshire.

Cantwell, J. (2015) *Leadership in Action*. Carlton, Vic.: Melbourne University Press.

Fitzsimons, P. (2012) *Batavia*. William Heineman. Random House Australia, North Sydney

Gentile, M.C. (2010) *Giving Voice to Values: How to Speak Your Mind When You Know What's Right*. New Haven, CT: Yale University Press.

George, B. (2003) *Authentic Leadership – Rediscovering the Secrets to Creating Lasting Value*. San Francisco: Jossey-Bass.

Hawking, S. (1988) *A Brief History of Time: From the Big Bang to Black Holes*. London: Bantam Books.

National Health Service Leadership Centre (2002) *NHS Leadership Qualities Framework*. London: NHS Leadership Centre.

Roberts, S.J. (1983) 'Oppressed group behaviour: implications for nursing', *Advances in Nursing Science*, 5: 21–30.

Stanley, D. (2004) 'Clinical leadership: a pilot study explored', *Paediatric Nursing*, 16 (3): 39–42.

Stanley, D. (2006a) 'Part 1: In command of care: clinical nurse leadership explored', *Journal of Research in Nursing*, II (1): 20–39.

Stanley, D. (2006b) 'Part 2: In command of care: towards the theory of congruent leadership', *Journal of Research in Nursing*, II (2): 132–44.

Stanley, D. (2006c) 'Recognising and defining clinical nurse leaders', *British Journal of Nursing*, 15 (2): 108–11.

Stanley, D. (2006d) 'Role conflict; leaders and managers', *Nursing Management*, 13 (5): 31–7.

Stanley, D. (2007) 'Lights in the shadows', *Contemporary Nurse*, 24 (1): 45–51.

Stanley, D. (2008) 'Congruent leadership: values in action', *Journal of Nursing Management*, 64: 84–95.

Stanley, D. (2009) 'Leadership: behind the mask', *ACORN*, 22 (1): 14–20.

Stanley, D. (2010) 'Clinical leadership and innovation', *Connections*, 13 (4): 27–8.

Stanley, D. (2011) *Clinical Leadership: Innovation into Action*. Melbourne: Palgrave Macmillan.

Stanley, D. (2012) 'Clinical leadership and innovation', *Journal of Nursing Education and Practice*, 2(2), 119–26.

Stanley, D. (2013a) Perceptions of Clinical Leadership in the St John Ambulance Service in WA: A Research Report. ISBN: 978-0-9875229-0-0 (Report). Accessed at http://www.sph.uwa.edu.au/__data/assets/pdf_file/0003/2272647/Report-Perceptions-of-clinical-leadership-in-the-St.pdf 1st December, 2018.

Stanley, D. (2014) 'Clinical leadership characteristics confirmed', *Journal of Research in Nursing*, 19 (2): 118—28.

Stanley, D. (2017) *Clinical Leadership in Nursing and Healthcare*. Oxford: Wiley Blackwell.

Stanley, D. and Sherratt, A. (2010) 'Lamp light on leadership: clinical leadership and Florence Nightingale', *Journal of Nursing Management*, 18: 115–21.

Stanley, D. and Stanley, K. (2017) 'Clinical leadership and Nursing Explored: A literature search, *Journal of Clinical Nursing*. 2018 May;27(9-10):1730-1743. doi: 10.1111/jocn.14145. Epub 2018 Jan 11. (DOI: 10.1111/jocn.14145 [epub ahead of print].

Stanley, D., Cuthbertson, J. and Latimer, K. (2012) 'Perceptions of clinical leadership in the St John Ambulance Service in WA: Paramedics Australasia', *Response*, 39 (1): 31–7.

Stanley, D., Hutton, M. and McDonald, A. (2015) Western Australian Allied Health Professionals' Perceptions of Clinical Leadership: A Research Report. Bathurst, NSW: CSU Print.

Stanley, D., Latimer, K. and Atkinson, J. (2014) 'Perceptions of clinical leadership in an aged care residential facility in Perth, Western Australia', Health Care Current Reviews, 2 (122). DOI: 10.4172/hccr.1000122.

Stanley, D., Blanchard, D., Holho, A., Hutton, M. and McDonald, A. (2017) 'Health Professionals' Perceptions of Clinical Leadership. A Pilot Study'. Cogent Medicine, 4. Available at: https://doi.org/10.1080/2331205X.2017.1321193

Wong, C. and Cummings, G. (2009) 'Authentic leadership: a new theory for nursing or back to basics?', *Journal of Health Organisations and Management*, 23 (5), 522 – 538.

CHAPTER 6

Antonakis, J., Ashkanasy, N. and Dasborough, M. (2009) 'Does leadership need emotional intelligence?', *Leadership Quarterly*, 20: 247–61.

Benson, G., Ploeg, J. and Brown, B. (2010) 'A cross-sectional study of emotional intelligence in baccalaureate nursing students', *Nurse Education Today*, 30: 49–53.

Brockbank, A. and McGill, I. (2007) *Facilitating Reflective Learning in Higher Education*. Buckingham: Open University Press.

Bulmer Smith, K., Profetto-McGrath, J. and Cummings, G. (2009) 'Emotional intelligence and nursing: an integrative literature review', *International Journal of Nursing Studies*, 46(12) 1624–36.

Chade-Meng, T. (2013) *Search Inside Yourself*. London: Collins.

Covey, S.R. (1989) *Seven Habits of Highly Effective People*. New York: Simon & Schuster.

Dillard, N.L. (1993) 'Development of hardiness', in Ann, Marriner–Tomey, *Transformational Leadership in Nursing*. St Louis, LA: Mosby Year Book.

Ebury, S. (1994) *Weary: The Life of Sir Edward Dunlop*. Ringwood: Viking.

Edwards, H. (2011) *Sir Edward 'Weary' Dunlop*. Frenchs Forest: New Frontier Publishing.

Gentile, M.C. (2010) *Giving Voice to Values*. New Haven, CT: Yale University Press.

Goleman, D. (1998) *Working with Emotional Intelligence*. New York: Bantam Books.

Goleman, D. (2005) *Emotional Intelligence*. New York: Bantam Books.

Goleman, D., Boyatzis, R. and McKee, A. (2013) *Primal Leadership: Unleashing the Power of Emotional Intelligence*. Boston: HBS Press.

Hall, C.S. and Lindzey, G. (1957) *Theories of Personality*, 1st edn. New York: Wiley.

Hawkes, R. (2017) *Telegraph*. Hacksaw Ridge: the extraordinary true story of Desmond Doss, the war hero who refused to kill. Available at: www.telegraph.co.uk/films/0/mel-gibsons-hacksaw-ridge-the-extraordinary-true-story-of-desmon/ (accessed 17 March 2018).

Heckemann, B., Schols, J. and Halfens, R. (2015) 'A reflective framework to foster emotionally intelligent leadership in nursing', *Journal of Nursing Management*, 23: 744–53.

Janowsky, D. S, Hong, E., Morter, S. & Howe, S (2002) Myers Briggs Type Indicator Personality Profiles in Unipolar Depressed Patients. November 2002, *The World Journal of Biological Psychiatry* 3(4):207-15. DOI:10.3109/15622970209150623

Kouzes, J.M. and Posner, B.Z. (2010) *The Truth About Leadership: The No-fads Heart of the Matter Facts You Need to Know*. San Francisco: Jossey-Bass.

Por, J., Barriball, L., Fitzpatrick, J. and Roberts, J. (2011) 'Emotional intelligence: its relationship to stress, coping, well-being and professional performance in nursing students', *Nurse Education Today*, 31:855–60.

Rajah, R., Song, Z. and Arvey, R. (2011) 'Emotionality and leadership: taking stock of the past decade of research', *Leadership Quarterly*, 22: 1107–19.

Rogers, C. (1979) *Carl Rogers on Personal Power*. New York: Delacorte.

Salovey, P. and Mayer. J. (1990) 'Emotional Intelligence', *Imagination, Cognition and Personality*, 9: 185–211.

Shakespeare, W. (1601) Hamlet, eds Ann Thompson and Neil Taylor (2006), *The Arden Shakespeare*, Third Series, 1. London: Cengage Learning.

Taylor, B., Roberts, S. and Smyth, T. (2015) 'Nurse managers' strategies for feeling less drained by their work: an action research and reflection project for developing emotional intelligence', *Journal of Nursing Management*, 23: 879–87.

Warren, H.C. and Carmichael, L. (1930) *Elements of Human Psychology*. Oxford: Houghton Mifflin.

Wiseman, T. (1996) 'A concept analysis of empathy', *Journal of Advanced Nursing*, 23 (6): 1162–7.

CHAPTER 7

Bickhoff, L. (2018) Changing the culture, one shift at a time. *The Hive*, Autumn 21, 10.

Brown, A. (1995) 'Organizational culture' (cited in S. Sun (2008), 'Organizational culture and its themes', *International Journal of Business and Management*, 3 (12): 137–41).

Cameron, K.S. and Quinn, R.E. (2011) *Diagnosing and Changing Organizational Culture*, 3rd edn. San Francisco: Jossey-Bass.

Chalmers, C, (2018) The nurse leader's role in workplace culture. *The Hive*, Autumn 21, 9.

Davies, H., Nutley, S.M. and Mannion, R. (2000) 'Organisational culture and quality in health care', *Quality in Health Care, 9* (1): 111–19.

Department of Health (UK) (2015) Culture Change in the NHS: Applying the Lessons of the Francis Inquiry. London: Stationery Office.

Dixon-Woods, M., Baker, R., Charles, K., Dawson, D., Jerzembek, G., Martin, G., McCarthy, I., McKee, L., Minion, J., Ozieranski, P., Wilkie, P. and West. M. (2013) Culture and Behaviour in the English National Health Service: Overview of Lessons from a Large Multimethod Study. *BMJ 'Quality and Safety First'*. 0:1-10 doi:10.1136/bmjqs-2013-001947

Fitz-Enz, J. (1997) *The 8 Practices of Exceptional Companies: How Great Organizations Make the Most of Their Human Assets*. New York: AMACOM.

Fowke, D. (1999) 'Shaping corporate culture', *New Management Network, 12* (2): 1–4. Available at: www.new-management-network.com/publications/Shaping%20 Corporate%20Culture.pdf

Francis, R. (2013) Report of the Mid Staffordshire NHS Foundation Trust Public Enquiry. London: Stationery Office.

Garvin, D. and Roberto, M. (2005) 'Reinforcing Values: A Public Dressing Down', *HBS Working Knowledge* [online], 14 March. Available at: hbswk.hbs.edu/item. jhtml?id=4688&t=leadership

Hall, M.L. (2005) 'Shaping organisational culture: a practitioner's perspective', Peak Development Consulting, 2 (1): 1–16.

Handy, C. (1999) *Understanding Organisations*, 3rd edn. London: Penguin Books.

Helmreich, R. and Merritt, A. (2005) *Culture at Work in Aviation and Medicine*. Burlington, VT: Ashgate.

Hofstede, G. and Bond, M.H. (1984) Hofstede's cultural dimensions: an independent validation using Rokeach's value survey', *Journal of Cross-cultural Psychology, 15* (4): 417–33.

Luthans, F., Norman, S.M., Avolio, B.M. and Avey, J. (2008) 'The mediating role of psychological capital in the supportive organisational climate – employee performance relationship', *Journal of Organisational Behavior*, 29: 219–38.

Neuhauser, P.C. (2005) 'Strategies for Changing Your Corporate Culture' [online]. Available at: www.culturedotcom.com/culturedotcom/article_4.htm

Orange Sky Australia. Available at: www.orangeskylaundry.com.au/?gclid=EAIaIQobChMI nMiFz82Q2QIVhQQqCh31rQXgEAAYASAAEgKySfD_BwE

Pink, D. (2009) *Drive: The Surprising Truth About What Motivates Us*. Riverhead Book, New York.

Rafferty, A.M., Philippou, J., Fitzpatrick, J.M. and Ball, J. (2015) *Culture of Care Barometer*, March. London: National Nursing Research Unit, Kings College London.

Rytterstrom, P., Unosson, M. and Arman, M. (2013) 'Care culture as a meaning-making process: a study of a mistreatment investigation', *Qualitative Health Research, 23* (9): 1179–87.

Schein, E.H. (2014) *Organizational Culture and Leadership*, 3rd edn. San Francisco: Jossey-Bass.

Scott, J.T., Mannion, R., Davies, H. and Marshall, M. (2003) 'The quantitative measurement of organizational culture in health care: what instruments are available?', *Health Service Research*, 38: 923–45.

Stanley, D. (2011) *Clinical Leadership: Innovation into Action*. South Yarra: Palgrave Macmillan.

Wei, Z., Baiyin, Y. and McLean, G.N. (2009) 'Linking organisational culture, structure, strategy and organisational effectiveness: mediating role of knowledge management', *Journal of Business Research, 63* (7): 763–71.

CHAPTER 8

Australian Banker Association (2013) Code of Banking Practice and Code of Compliance Monitoring Committee Mandate. Australian Bankers Association Inc.

Bickhoff, L. (2018) 'Changing the culture, one shift at a time', *The Hive*, 21: 10.

Chalmers, C. (2018) 'The nurse leader's role in workplace culture', *The Hive*, 21: 9.

Hall, M.L. (2005) 'Shaping organisational culture: a practitioner's perspective', Peak Development Consulting, 2 (1): 1–16.

Horwitz, T. (2011) *Midnight Rising*. New York: Picador.

Johns Hopkins School of Nursing (2017) 'Editorial', February. Available at: https://magazine.nursing.jhu.edu/2017/02/moral-distress-and-building-resilience/

CHAPTER 9

Bostridge, M. (2004) 'The ladies with the lamps', *BBC History*, 18–19 October.

Bostridge, M. (2008) *Florence Nightingale: The Woman and Her Legend*. London: Viking.

Cornwell, B. (2014) *Waterloo: The History of Four Days, Three Armies and Three Battles*. London: William Collins.

Courtenay, B. (2007) *A Recipe for Dreaming*. Camberwell, Victoria Australia: Viking.

Guelzo, A.C. (2014) *Gettysburg: The Last Invasion*. New York: First Vintage Books Edition.

Keegan, J. (1996). *The Face of Battle: A Study of Agincourt, Waterloo and the Somme*. London: Pimlico.

Pondy, L.R. (1978) 'Leadership is a language game', in M.W. McCall Jr and M.M. Lombardo (eds), *Leadership: Where Else Can We Go?* Durham, NC: Duke University Press.

Reed, R. (2018) *If I Could Tell You Just One Thing …* Edinburgh: Canongate Books.

Woodham-Smith, C. (1982) *Florence Nightingale*. London: Constable.

INDEX